Retrain Your Sleep Brain

Evidence-Based CBT-I Strategies to End Chronic Insomnia, Stop Sleep Anxiety, and Restore Natural Patterns Without Medication

Hades Kishi Whitaker

First Edition

Paperback: ISBN: 978-1-923604-64-3

eBook ISBN: 978-1-923604-65-0

Table of Contents

Introduction: Reclaiming Your Sleep

It's 3 AM. Again.

You might be staring at the ceiling, watching the shadows on the wall, or maybe you're anxiously checking the clock. You're calculating how little sleep you'll get if you fall asleep *right now*. The house is quiet, the world outside is still, but your mind? It's racing. If you've experienced nights like this—nights filled with frustration, worry, and a desperate wish for rest—believe me, you are certainly not alone.

Living without enough sleep is hard. It's more than just feeling tired during the day. It affects everything. Your mood, your energy, your ability to think clearly, even your physical health. It can feel like you're walking through life in a fog, never quite fully present. Maybe you're irritable with your family (we've all been there), struggling to focus at work, or you've stopped doing things you enjoy because you simply don't have the energy.

This workbook is designed to help you change that. Now, look, this isn't filled with quick fixes, magic pills, or promises of perfect sleep every single night. Instead, it offers something much better: a set of tools and strategies proven by science to help you understand why you aren't sleeping and how to fix it for the long term. We are going to tackle the root causes of your insomnia, not just the symptoms.

If you're reading this, you've likely already tried many things. Maybe herbal teas, melatonin, blackout curtains, strict routines. Maybe even medications. And yet, the sleep problem persists. This can be incredibly discouraging. You might start to believe that you are just a "bad sleeper" or that nothing will ever work.

Here's the good news: Insomnia is highly treatable. And the approach we will use in this workbook is the most effective treatment available today.

Understanding the impact of insomnia

Insomnia isn't just a nighttime problem; it's a 24-hour problem. When we talk about insomnia, we mean more than just having a bad night here and there. Everyone sleeps poorly sometimes, especially when stressed. *Chronic insomnia*, however, is different. It means having trouble falling asleep, staying asleep, or waking up too early at least three nights a week, for three months or longer (American Psychiatric Association, 2013).

The effects of this ongoing sleep loss ripple through every aspect of life.

Mentally and Emotionally:

You probably notice it's harder to concentrate. Making decisions feels difficult, and your memory might not be as sharp. Emotionally, the lack of sleep can make you feel anxious, depressed, or just generally irritable. It's like the volume knob on all your difficult emotions gets turned way up. Small stressors? They feel like big crises. Research consistently shows a strong link between chronic insomnia and an increased risk of developing mental health conditions like depression and anxiety disorders (Baglioni et al., 2011).

Physically:

Sleep is when our bodies repair themselves. Without enough quality sleep, our physical health suffers. Chronic insomnia has been linked to a host of physical problems. It can weaken your immune system, making it harder to fight off common illnesses. It's also associated with a higher risk of long-term health issues, including high blood pressure, heart disease, and diabetes (Institute of Medicine, 2006). It can also mess with your metabolism and make it harder to maintain a healthy weight.

Socially and Professionally:

When you're exhausted, you might withdraw. You cancel plans because you're too tired, or maybe you're there physically but zoned out mentally. At work, productivity often drops. You might make more mistakes. In some jobs, the drowsiness can even be dangerous, especially if you drive frequently.

The frustration of not being able to sleep often leads to a deep sense of isolation. It feels like everyone else can do this simple, natural thing—sleep—but you can't. Understanding the broad impact of insomnia is the first step toward recognizing why it's so important to treat it effectively. This isn't just about feeling less tired; it's about improving your quality of life.

Introduction to Cognitive Behavioral Therapy for Insomnia (CBT-I) as the gold-standard treatment

So, what is the most effective way to treat chronic insomnia? You might be surprised to learn that it's not sleeping pills. While medications can offer short-term relief, they don't address the underlying causes. They are a band-aid. Over time, they can become less effective, and some can be habit-forming.

The leading treatment, recommended as the first line of defense by major medical organizations like the American College of Physicians, is Cognitive Behavioral Therapy for Insomnia, or CBT-I (Qaseem et al., 2016).

What exactly is CBT-I? It sounds technical, but it's actually very practical. CBT-I is a structured program that helps you identify and replace the thoughts and behaviors that are causing or worsening your sleep problems with habits that promote sound sleep. Unlike medication, CBT-I helps you develop skills that last a lifetime.

Let's break it down:

- **Cognitive:** This refers to your thoughts and beliefs about sleep. If you lie in bed worrying about the consequences of not sleeping, your mind becomes active and alert. This anxiety makes sleep even harder to achieve. CBT-I helps you challenge these unhelpful thoughts.

- **Behavioral:** This refers to your actions and habits. Many people with insomnia develop behaviors that actually interfere with sleep. For example, spending too much time in bed awake, or trying to force sleep. CBT-I teaches you healthy behaviors that help your body regulate its natural sleep mechanisms.

CBT-I is powerful because it addresses the *perpetuating factors* of insomnia—the things you might be doing (often unintentionally) that keep the insomnia going long after the initial trigger has passed.

How effective is it? Very. Research shows that CBT-I works as well as, or even better than, sleep medication in the short term, and significantly better in the long term. Studies indicate that 70% to 80% of people with chronic insomnia see significant improvements after completing CBT-I (Morin et al., 1999). Many find they can reduce or eliminate their need for sleep medications entirely.

CBT-I puts you back in control. Instead of sleep being something unpredictable that happens to you, you will learn how to create the conditions that allow sleep to happen naturally.

How this workbook is structured

(the 6-8 week journey)

This workbook is designed to guide you through the core components of CBT-I step by step. It's structured much like a course you might take with a sleep specialist. The program typically takes about 6 to 8 weeks.

It's important to follow the workbook in order. Each section builds on the skills learned in the previous ones. Think of it like building a house. You need a solid foundation before you can start putting up the walls.

Here is a roadmap of our journey together:

Part 1: Foundations of Sleep and Insomnia (Weeks 1-2)

We will start by understanding how sleep works and what causes insomnia. This knowledge is crucial because it helps you understand why we are asking you to make certain changes. We will also begin the important task of tracking your sleep using a daily sleep diary. This baseline information is essential.

Part 2: Behavioral Strategies - Retraining Your Body to Sleep (Weeks 3-5)

This is where we introduce the most powerful behavioral techniques: Stimulus Control and Sleep Restriction. These strategies are designed to break the association between your bed and wakefulness, and to build up a strong, consistent sleep drive. These techniques can be challenging at first—I won't lie—but they are often the key to unlocking deep, restorative sleep.

Part 3: Cognitive Strategies - Calming Your Mind (Weeks 5-6)

Once we have addressed the behaviors, we will focus on the cognitive aspects. We will tackle the worry, frustration, and unhelpful beliefs that interfere with sleep. You will learn techniques for cognitive restructuring to change your relationship with sleep and reduce nighttime anxiety.

Part 4: Lifestyle and Relaxation (Week 7)

We will look at how your daily habits and routines affect your sleep. This includes sleep hygiene—optimizing your environment and lifestyle choices. We will also introduce various relaxation techniques to help you wind down.

Part 5: Maintaining Progress and Troubleshooting (Week 8+)

Finally, we will focus on making these changes stick. We will discuss how to handle setbacks (they will happen!) and develop a long-term plan for maintaining healthy sleep.

This is not just reading. It's an active process of learning and change.

The importance of commitment and realistic expectations

Starting a CBT-I program requires commitment. You will be asked to make significant changes to your habits, and some of these changes might feel difficult or counterintuitive at first. Here's the thing: There might be times when you feel *more* tired before you start feeling better. This is a normal part of the process as your body adjusts to a new sleep schedule.

Think of it like starting a new exercise program. If you haven't run in years, your first few jogs will be uncomfortable. But if you stick with it, your body adapts, and it gets easier. The same is true for retraining your sleep system.

Here are some key principles for success:

1. Be Patient and Persistent:

CBT-I is not an overnight fix. It takes time to change ingrained habits and thought patterns. Don't get discouraged if you don't see immediate results. Consistency is key. Sticking with the program, even on tough days, is essential for long-term success.

2. Be Honest with Yourself:

Accurate self-monitoring is crucial. When you fill out your sleep diaries, be as honest and accurate as possible. You are doing this work for yourself, and the effectiveness of the program depends on having good data.

3. Set Realistic Expectations:

The goal of CBT-I is not necessarily to achieve perfect sleep every night. Even the best sleepers have occasional bad nights. The goal is to improve the quality of your sleep, reduce the distress caused by insomnia, and improve your daytime functioning. We are aiming for progress, not perfection.

4. Embrace the Challenge:

6

Change is hard, but living with chronic insomnia is harder. Embrace the challenges of the program as opportunities for growth. You are taking active steps to improve your health and well-being.

Starting this journey is a significant step. By committing to this process, you are investing in yourself. You have the capacity to sleep well. This workbook will provide you with the tools you need to unlock that capacity. Let's begin the process of reclaiming your sleep.

Chapter 1: The Science of Sleep

To fix a problem, you first need to understand it. If your car breaks down, a mechanic needs to understand how the engine works before they can figure out what's wrong. Right? The same is true for sleep. Many people with insomnia have misunderstandings about how sleep actually works, and these misunderstandings can actually make the problem worse.

If you believe you need exactly eight hours of sleep to function, you'll become anxious when you only get six. If you don't understand your body clock, you might try to sleep at the wrong times. This chapter is about laying the groundwork. We're going to explore the biology of sleep in a simple, straightforward way. Understanding the science behind sleep will help you see why the strategies in this workbook are so effective.

Sleep is not just a period of inactivity. It's a dynamic and essential process. It used to be thought that the brain simply shut down during sleep. But research has shown that the brain is actually quite active during sleep, carrying out critical maintenance and restoration tasks.

Why we sleep: The functions of sleep

Why do we spend nearly a third of our lives asleep? It must be important, right? Absolutely. Sleep serves many vital functions across the entire body. When you don't get enough quality sleep, these functions are impaired.

Here are some of the main reasons why sleep is so crucial:

1. Brain Maintenance and Memory Consolidation:

While you sleep, your brain is busy processing the information you learned during the day. It organizes memories, strengthens important connections between brain cells, and trims away the unnecessary stuff. This process, known as memory consolidation, is essential for learning. If you've ever tried to study for a test, you know how important a good night's sleep is for making that information stick (Rasch & Born, 2013).

Furthermore, recent research has shown that sleep helps clear waste products from the brain. Think of it like a nightly cleaning crew. During the day, as your brain cells work hard, they produce metabolic waste, including proteins linked to diseases like Alzheimer's. While you sleep, the flow of fluid in the brain increases, washing away these harmful substances (Xie et al., 2013). This detoxification process is vital for long-term brain health.

2. Physical Restoration and Repair:

Sleep is a time for the body to heal. During deep sleep, the body releases growth hormone, which is essential for cell growth, muscle repair, and tissue regeneration. If you've had a hard workout or an injury, sleep is critical for recovery. This helps explain why you feel physically rundown when you are sleep-deprived.

3. Immune System Support:

Sleep plays a key role in regulating your immune system. While you sleep, your body produces proteins called cytokines, which help fight inflammation and infection. When you don't get enough sleep, the production of these protective cytokines decreases, making you more vulnerable to illness. Studies have shown that people who consistently sleep poorly are more likely to get sick after being exposed to a virus, such as the common cold (Cohen et al., 2009).

4. Emotional Regulation:

Have you ever noticed how much harder it is to manage your emotions when you're tired? You feel more irritable, anxious, or sad. Sleep is essential for emotional balance. During sleep, particularly REM sleep (which we'll discuss shortly), the brain processes emotional experiences. When you are sleep-deprived, the emotional centers of the brain become more reactive to negative stimuli. A good night's sleep helps reset your emotional thermostat.

5. Metabolic and Cardiovascular Health:

Sleep helps regulate your metabolism—how your body uses energy. Chronic sleep deprivation can affect how your body processes glucose, increasing the risk of type 2 diabetes. It also affects the hormones that control hunger, which can lead to weight gain. Furthermore, sleep is important for cardiovascular health. During deep sleep, your heart rate and blood pressure decrease, giving your cardiovascular system a chance to rest.

In short, sleep is not a luxury; it's a fundamental biological need, just like eating, drinking, and breathing. Understanding this helps shift the perspective from seeing sleep as an inconvenience to recognizing it as a critical pillar of health.

The architecture of sleep: NREM and REM cycles

Sleep is not uniform. It doesn't just turn on and off like a light switch. Instead, we move through different stages of sleep throughout the night in a predictable pattern known as the *sleep cycle*. This structure is called *sleep architecture*.

There are two main types of sleep:

1. **NREM (Non-Rapid Eye Movement) Sleep:** This is further divided into three stages (N1, N2, and N3).

2. **REM (Rapid Eye Movement) Sleep:** This is when most vivid dreaming occurs.

Let's look at what happens in each stage:

NREM Stage 1 (N1): The Gateway to Sleep

This is the lightest stage. It's the transition between wakefulness and sleep. Your brain waves, heart rate, and eye movements begin to slow down. Your muscles start to relax. This stage usually lasts only a few minutes. You can be easily awakened. Sometimes you might experience sudden muscle jerks or that weird sensation of falling.

NREM Stage 2 (N2): Light Sleep

You are now asleep, but it's still relatively light. Your heart rate and breathing slow down even more, and your body temperature drops slightly. The brain waves continue to slow, but with occasional bursts of rapid waves called sleep spindles and structures called K-complexes. We spend about half the night in N2 sleep.

NREM Stage 3 (N3): Deep Sleep (Slow-Wave Sleep)

This is the deepest stage of sleep, also known as slow-wave sleep because of the slow delta brain waves that occur. It is much harder to wake someone up from N3 sleep, and if you are awakened, you will likely feel groggy and disoriented for a few minutes (this is called sleep inertia).

Deep sleep is crucial for physical restoration. This is when the body repairs tissues, builds bone and muscle, and strengthens the immune system. Deep sleep is essential for feeling refreshed and energetic in the morning.

REM Sleep (R): The Dreaming Stage

After deep sleep, you cycle back up to lighter sleep and then enter REM sleep. This stage is fascinating. As the name suggests, your eyes move rapidly from side to side behind closed eyelids. Your brain activity increases, almost to the level seen when you are awake.

REM sleep is when most of our vivid, story-like dreams occur. While the brain is highly active, the muscles in your arms and legs become temporarily paralyzed. This is a protective mechanism to prevent you from acting out your dreams (thank goodness!).

REM sleep is particularly important for cognitive functions like memory processing and emotional regulation.

The Sleep Cycle:

Throughout the night, we cycle through these stages. A complete sleep cycle lasts about 90 to 120 minutes. Most adults complete 4 to 6 cycles per night.

The composition of the cycles changes as the night progresses. In the first half of the night, we get more deep sleep (N3). In the second half of the night, the proportion of REM sleep increases.

Here's a typical pattern:

Wake → N1 → N2 → N3 → N2 → REM

Understanding sleep architecture is important. If you have trouble falling asleep, you are struggling to transition through N1 and N2. If you wake up frequently, you might be experiencing disruptions in the normal progression of the cycles. If you wake up feeling unrefreshed, you might not be getting enough deep sleep (N3) or REM sleep.

Many factors can disrupt sleep architecture, including stress, age (we tend to get less deep sleep as we get older), alcohol, and certain medications. The strategies in this workbook are designed to help restore a more natural and healthy sleep pattern.

The two drivers of sleep

What makes us fall asleep? It's not just about feeling tired at the end of the day. Our sleep-wake cycle is regulated by two main biological mechanisms. These two systems work together to determine when we sleep and when we wake up.

1. Homeostatic Sleep Drive (The Need for Sleep)

This is often called *sleep pressure* or *sleep drive*. It's a very simple concept: the longer you stay awake, the sleepier you become.

Imagine sleep drive as a balloon filling up with water. From the moment you wake up, the balloon starts filling. The longer you are awake, the more water goes into the balloon, and the higher the pressure becomes. When the pressure reaches a certain point, you feel a strong urge to sleep.

When you sleep, the balloon drains. The longer and deeper you sleep, the more the pressure is released. When you wake up in the morning, the balloon is empty, and you feel refreshed.

This process is driven by the accumulation of certain chemicals in the brain, most notably a substance called *adenosine*. Adenosine builds up throughout the day, promoting sleepiness. When you sleep, adenosine is cleared away.

By the way, caffeine works by blocking the effects of adenosine. It temporarily masks your sleep drive. But the adenosine is still building up. When the caffeine wears off? Crash. You feel a sudden wave of sleepiness as the accumulated sleep pressure hits you.

Understanding sleep drive is crucial for treating insomnia. Many of the strategies in CBT-I are designed to increase your homeostatic sleep drive before bed. For example:

- **Waking up at a consistent time:** This ensures that your sleep drive starts building at the same time every day.

- **Avoiding naps:** Napping during the day releases some of the sleep pressure, making it harder to fall asleep at night. It's like letting some water out of the balloon prematurely.

- **Sleep Restriction Therapy (which we will discuss later):** This technique intentionally limits the time spent in bed to build up a stronger sleep drive, leading to more consolidated sleep.

If you lie in bed awake for hours, you are not effectively building sleep drive. You might feel tired, but you are not necessarily *sleepy* in a way that promotes deep sleep.

2. The Circadian Rhythm (The Internal Body Clock)

The second system is the *circadian rhythm*. This is your internal biological clock, located in the brain. This clock regulates various bodily processes over a roughly 24-hour cycle, including body temperature, hormone release, and, most importantly, your sleep-wake cycle.

The word "circadian" means "about a day."

The circadian rhythm acts as an alerting signal. It promotes wakefulness during the day and allows sleepiness to take over at night. It's what makes you feel alert in the morning and sleepy in the evening.

Think of the circadian rhythm as the conductor of an orchestra, keeping all the different bodily systems synchronized.

The most important external cue that helps synchronize your internal clock is light. Exposure to bright light during the day, especially in the morning, strengthens the circadian rhythm and promotes alertness. Light exposure at night, particularly blue light from electronic devices (phones, tablets), can disrupt the circadian rhythm by suppressing the release of *melatonin*, a hormone that signals to the body that it's time to sleep.

Your circadian rhythm is not exactly 24 hours. It tends to be slightly longer. This is why we need external cues (like light and meals) to keep it aligned with the 24-hour day.

How the Two Systems Interact:

The interaction between the sleep drive and the circadian rhythm determines your level of alertness.

The sleep drive builds steadily throughout the day. The circadian alerting signal increases during the day, helping to counteract the rising sleep drive, and then drops off in the evening.

The ideal time for sleep is when the sleep drive is high and the circadian alerting signal is low. This typically occurs in the late evening.

In the morning, the sleep drive is low, and the circadian alerting signal increases, promoting wakefulness.

Understanding this interaction helps explain certain phenomena:

- **The afternoon dip:** You might notice a dip in alertness in the early afternoon (around 2-4 PM). This is because the circadian alerting signal temporarily decreases slightly, while the sleep drive continues to build.

- **The "second wind":** Sometimes, if you stay up past your usual bedtime, you might get a burst of energy. This is because your circadian rhythm is starting to promote wakefulness again, even though your sleep drive is high.

- **Jet lag:** When you travel across time zones, your internal clock is out of sync with the local time. It takes time for your internal clock to adjust.

Insomnia often involves a misalignment of these two systems. CBT-I strategies aim to synchronize them by promoting a strong sleep drive and stabilizing the circadian rhythm through consistent schedules and healthy habits.

How much sleep do you really need? Dispelling common sleep myths

One of the biggest sources of anxiety for people with insomnia is the belief that they need a specific amount of sleep to function well. We are constantly told about the importance of getting eight hours. But the truth is, sleep needs vary.

The Myth of the Eight-Hour Requirement:

The idea that everyone needs eight hours of sleep is a myth. Sleep needs are individual and influenced by genetics, age, and activity level. The National Sleep Foundation recommends that most adults get between 7 and 9 hours of sleep per night (Hirshkowitz et al., 2015). However, some people are naturally *short sleepers* who function perfectly well on 6 hours, while others are *long sleepers* who need 10 hours.

The important question is not "How many hours did I sleep?" but rather "How do I feel during the day?" If you feel refreshed and alert most of the day, you are probably getting enough sleep, even if it's less than eight hours.

Worrying about getting a certain number of hours can actually make insomnia worse. If you lie in bed calculating how much sleep you've lost, you create anxiety and arousal that interfere with sleep. This is called *sleep performance anxiety*.

Common Sleep Myths:

Let's look at some other common myths about sleep that can contribute to insomnia:

Myth 1: If I don't sleep well one night, I won't be able to function the next day.

Fact: While you might not feel your best after a bad night's sleep, you can usually function reasonably well. Your body compensates for short-term sleep loss. Believing that your day will be ruined can create a self-fulfilling prophecy. If you expect to feel terrible, you probably will.

Myth 2: I need to catch up on lost sleep on the weekends.

Fact: Trying to compensate by sleeping in late on the weekends can disrupt your circadian rhythm and make insomnia worse. This pattern, known as social jetlag, confuses your internal clock. It's like flying across time zones every weekend. The best approach is to maintain a consistent sleep schedule, including a regular wake-up time, seven days a week.

Myth 3: If I wake up in the middle of the night, I should stay in bed and try to fall back asleep.

Fact: Waking up during the night is normal. Even good sleepers wake up briefly several times a night as they transition between sleep cycles. They usually fall back asleep quickly and don't remember it. If you find yourself awake for more than 15-20 minutes, staying in

16

bed and trying to force sleep leads to frustration. This trains your brain to associate the bed with wakefulness. It's better to get out of bed. (We will cover this later in Stimulus Control).

Myth 4: Alcohol helps you sleep.

Fact: While alcohol can make you drowsy and help you fall asleep faster, it disrupts the quality of your sleep. Alcohol suppresses REM sleep early on. As it wears off, you experience fragmented and shallow sleep in the second half of the night. You wake up feeling unrefreshed.

Myth 5: Napping during the day is a good way to make up for lost sleep.

Fact: For people with insomnia, daytime napping can make it harder to sleep at night. Napping reduces your homeostatic sleep drive (it drains the sleep pressure balloon). If you must nap, keep it short (20-30 minutes) and early in the afternoon. However, during the initial stages of CBT-I, it is generally recommended to avoid napping altogether.

Understanding the science of sleep and debunking these common myths is a powerful first step. It allows you to let go of unrealistic expectations and focus on the strategies that actually work.

A Look Back at Sleep Science

- **Sleep is essential:** It's not just inactivity. Sleep is critical for brain maintenance, physical restoration, immune support, emotional regulation, and overall health.

- **Sleep has structure:** We cycle through different stages (NREM light sleep, NREM deep sleep, and REM sleep) throughout the night.

- **Two systems drive sleep:** The homeostatic sleep drive (sleep pressure) builds up the longer you are awake. The circadian rhythm (internal body clock) regulates the timing of sleep and wakefulness.

- **Sleep needs are individual:** There is no magic number of hours everyone needs. Worrying about the clock can worsen insomnia.

- **Myths can harm sleep:** Believing common misconceptions about sleep can lead to behaviors and attitudes that interfere with healthy sleep.

Chapter 2: Understanding Your Insomnia

Now that we've covered how sleep is supposed to work, let's talk about what happens when it doesn't. Insomnia is complex. It's usually not just one thing going wrong. It typically involves a combination of factors that interact to create and maintain sleep problems.

Understanding the nature of your insomnia—what type you have, what might have triggered it, and, crucially, what is keeping it going—is essential for developing an effective treatment plan. This chapter will help you become a detective of your own sleep patterns. We will explore how short-term sleep issues can morph into long-term chronic insomnia.

We will also look at the vicious cycle of insomnia, anxiety, and arousal that often keeps people trapped. By the end of this chapter, you should have a clearer understanding of the factors contributing to your sleep difficulties.

Types of insomnia (difficulty falling asleep, staying asleep, waking too early)

Insomnia is not a one-size-fits-all condition. It can manifest in different ways. Understanding your specific pattern can help tailor the treatment.

Here are the main ways insomnia presents:

1. Sleep-Onset Insomnia (Difficulty Falling Asleep)

This means having trouble initiating sleep at the beginning of the night. You might lie in bed for 30 minutes or longer before falling asleep. This is often associated with anxiety, worry, a racing mind, or a delayed circadian rhythm (being a "night owl"). You might feel tired during the day, but when you get into bed? Boom. Your mind suddenly becomes active and alert.

Case Example: Sarah

Sarah always considered herself a worrier. When she went to bed at 10:30 PM, her mind would immediately start reviewing the day's events and planning for tomorrow. She would worry about work deadlines, family issues, and, eventually, the fact that she wasn't falling asleep. She would toss and turn, check the clock, and feel increasingly frustrated. It often took her over an hour to finally drift off.

2. Sleep-Maintenance Insomnia (Difficulty Staying Asleep)

This involves waking up frequently during the night and having trouble falling back asleep. You might fall asleep easily at first, but then find yourself awake multiple times. These awakenings can last minutes or hours.

This can be caused by various factors, including medical conditions (like pain or sleep apnea), environmental disturbances (noise, light), alcohol consumption, or simply the learned habit of being awake in the middle of the night.

Case Example: Mark

Mark usually fell asleep quickly around 11 PM. But he consistently woke up around 2 AM. Sometimes he needed to use the bathroom, but other times he woke up for no apparent reason. Once awake, he would start thinking about his job stress. He would lie in bed trying to force himself back to sleep, but the more he tried, the more awake he felt. He would often stay awake for an hour or two.

3. Early Morning Awakening (Waking Up Too Early)

This means waking up earlier than desired and being unable to fall back asleep. For example, waking up at 4 AM when your alarm is set for 7 AM. This is often associated with depression, anxiety, or an advanced circadian rhythm. It can also be related to age, as our sleep patterns tend to shift earlier as we get older.

Case Example: Maria

Maria, in her late 50s, started waking up consistently at 4:30 AM. She wanted to sleep until 6 AM, but no matter what time she went to bed, she would wake up early. Once awake, she felt tired but unable to return to sleep.

Mixed Insomnia:

Many people experience a combination of these patterns.

Acute vs. Chronic Insomnia:

It's also important to distinguish between acute and chronic insomnia.

- *Acute insomnia* (short-term) is brief, usually lasting a few days or weeks. It is often triggered by a specific stressful event—a job interview, an illness, or a change in routine. Acute insomnia is very common. It usually resolves on its own when the stressor passes.

- *Chronic insomnia* is long-term. It is defined as having trouble sleeping at least three nights a week for three months or longer (American Psychiatric Association, 2013). Chronic insomnia often starts as acute insomnia, but it persists long after the initial trigger is gone. This is where the "3P" model comes in.

The "3P" Model of Insomnia

The "3P" model, developed by Dr. Arthur Spielman, is a widely accepted framework for understanding how chronic insomnia develops (Spielman et al., 1987). It suggests that insomnia is influenced by three types of factors: Predisposing, Precipitating, and Perpetuating.

Imagine a threshold for insomnia. If the combination of these factors pushes you above this threshold, you will experience sleep difficulties.

1. Predisposing factors (what makes you vulnerable)

These are factors that make you more likely to develop insomnia. They are present before the insomnia begins. They don't cause the insomnia directly, but they increase your vulnerability. Think of them as the background setting.

Predisposing factors can include:

- **Genetics:** Some people are biologically predisposed to being lighter sleepers or having a more reactive sleep system.

- **Personality Traits:** Certain traits, such as perfectionism, a tendency to worry, or difficulty relaxing, can make you more prone to insomnia.

- **Hyperarousal:** Some people have a higher level of physiological arousal—their bodies and minds are generally more "revved up." This heightened state of alertness can interfere with the ability to wind down.

- **Age and Gender:** Insomnia becomes more common with age, and women are more likely to experience it than men.

Having predisposing factors doesn't mean you are destined to have insomnia. It just means you might have a lower threshold for developing sleep problems when stress occurs.

2. Precipitating factors (what triggered it)

These are the events or circumstances that trigger the onset of insomnia. They are the immediate causes of the sleep disruption. Precipitating factors usually lead to acute insomnia.

Common precipitating factors include:

- **Stress:** This is one of the most common triggers. Job loss, financial difficulties, relationship problems, or grief can disrupt sleep.

- **Medical Illness:** Physical health problems, such as pain, hormonal imbalances, or respiratory issues.

- **Mental Health Conditions:** Anxiety disorders, depression, PTSD.

- **Medications:** Some medications can interfere with sleep.

- **Changes in Routine or Environment:** Jet lag, shift work, or a new baby.

In many cases, the precipitating factor is clear. You know exactly when and why your sleep problems started.

3. Perpetuating factors (what keeps it going) – the focus of CBT-I

This is the most crucial part of the model for understanding chronic insomnia. Perpetuating factors are the thoughts and behaviors that maintain the sleep problem long after the initial precipitating factor has resolved.

When people experience acute insomnia, they often try to cope in ways that make sense at the time but actually backfire in the long run. These coping strategies become the habits that perpetuate the insomnia.

Common perpetuating factors include:

- **Spending too much time in bed awake:** In an effort to get more sleep, people might go to bed earlier or stay in bed later. This weakens the association between the bed and sleep, training the brain to associate the bed with wakefulness and frustration.

- **Irregular sleep schedules:** Sleeping in on weekends or having inconsistent bedtimes disrupts the circadian rhythm.

- **Worrying about sleep (Sleep Anxiety):** Worrying about the consequences of not sleeping creates arousal that interferes with sleep.

- **Trying too hard to sleep (Sleep Effort):** Trying to force sleep creates tension and alertness that prevent sleep from occurring. The effort itself becomes the barrier.

- **Unhelpful beliefs about sleep:** Holding onto myths (e.g., "I must have 8 hours") increases anxiety.

How the 3P Model Explains Chronic Insomnia:

Let's look at how these factors interact using a case example.

Case Example: David

David was always a somewhat light sleeper and a bit of a worrier (**Predisposing factors**). A few months ago, his company announced layoffs, and he became very stressed about his job security (**Precipitating factor**). He started having trouble falling asleep because his mind was racing.

To cope, David started going to bed earlier. He also started sleeping in on weekends. When he couldn't sleep, he would stay in bed and watch TV or look at his phone. He started worrying about his insomnia, fearing it would affect his performance at work.

Eventually, David's job situation stabilized. The stress passed. But the insomnia continued. Why? Because his coping strategies had become **Perpetuating factors**. He had trained his brain to associate his bed with wakefulness and anxiety. His irregular schedule disrupted his internal clock. His worry about sleep created a vicious cycle.

The original trigger (job stress) was gone, but the insomnia had taken on a life of its own.

The Focus of CBT-I:

CBT-I focuses primarily on addressing the perpetuating factors. We cannot change your predisposing factors (your genetics). We cannot change the precipitating factors (the past stress). But we **can** change the thoughts and behaviors that are currently maintaining your sleep problems. This is the key.

By targeting the perpetuating factors, CBT-I breaks the cycle of chronic insomnia.

The vicious cycle of insomnia, anxiety, and arousal

One of the most frustrating aspects of insomnia is the vicious cycle of anxiety and arousal that often develops. When sleep becomes a struggle, it's natural to feel anxious about it. But this anxiety itself makes sleep even harder to achieve.

Let's break down how this cycle works.

1. The Trigger: A Bad Night's Sleep

It starts with a period of poor sleep. You have trouble falling or staying asleep, and you feel tired the next day.

2. The Reaction: Worry and Anxiety

Because sleep is essential, you naturally become concerned. You start having thoughts like:

- "If I don't fall asleep soon, I won't be able to function tomorrow."

- "This is ruining my health."

- "Why can't I sleep like a normal person?"

These thoughts create anxiety and frustration.

3. The Consequence: Increased Arousal

Anxiety triggers the body's stress response (the "fight-or-flight" response). Your heart rate increases, your muscles tense up, and your mind becomes alert. This state of hyperarousal is the exact opposite of what you need to fall asleep. Sleep requires a calm mind and a relaxed body.

4. The Result: More Sleep Difficulty

When you are aroused, it is much harder to fall asleep. You might lie in bed feeling wired but tired. The longer you stay awake, the more anxious you become, which further increases arousal.

5. The Cycle Continues: Conditioned Arousal

Over time, this cycle can lead to conditioned arousal. Your brain starts to associate your bed and bedtime with anxiety and wakefulness. Even if you are tired before getting into bed, as soon as you lie down, you might suddenly feel wide awake. The bed itself becomes a cue for arousal.

Think of it like this: If you spend night after night in bed feeling anxious and frustrated, you will start to feel anxious and frustrated just being in bed.

The Role of Sleep Effort:

Another factor that feeds this vicious cycle is *sleep effort*. When you are desperate for sleep, you try hard to make it happen. You try to force your mind to be quiet, or engage in elaborate rituals to induce sleep.

But sleep is not something you can actively control. It's an involuntary process, like breathing. Trying to force sleep is like trying to force yourself to feel happy. It doesn't work, and it usually creates more tension.

As Dr. Colin Espie, a leading expert in sleep medicine, puts it:

"The harder you try to sleep, the less likely you are to succeed." (Espie, 2006)

The effort to sleep sends a message to your brain that there is a problem that needs to be solved. This activates the problem-solving centers of your brain, making sleep even more elusive.

Breaking the Cycle:

CBT-I is designed to break this vicious cycle at multiple points.

- **Behavioral Strategies (Stimulus Control and Sleep Restriction):** These techniques help break the conditioned association between the bed and arousal. By getting out of bed when you can't sleep, you stop reinforcing the connection between the bed and frustration.

- **Cognitive Strategies (Cognitive Restructuring):** These techniques help you challenge the unhelpful thoughts and beliefs that fuel anxiety.

- **Relaxation Techniques:** These strategies help you reduce physiological arousal by calming your body and mind.

By understanding the mechanisms that maintain your insomnia, you can start to dismantle them. Recognizing that your insomnia is perpetuated by factors you can control is empowering. It means you are not helpless. You have the ability to change your habits and thought patterns and reclaim your sleep.

In the next chapter, we will start the process of assessing your sleep patterns and setting goals. This will provide the baseline information we need to tailor the CBT-I strategies to your specific needs.

Understanding Insomnia Insights

- **Insomnia takes different forms:** It can involve difficulty falling asleep (sleep-onset), staying asleep (sleep-maintenance), or waking up too early (early morning awakening).

- **Acute vs. Chronic:** Acute insomnia is short-term and usually triggered by stress. Chronic insomnia is long-term and persists after the trigger is gone.

- **The 3P Model explains development:** Predisposing factors make you vulnerable. Precipitating factors trigger the onset. Perpetuating factors (thoughts and behaviors) maintain the problem.

- **CBT-I targets perpetuating factors:** The focus is on changing the habits and attitudes that keep insomnia going.

- **The vicious cycle of anxiety:** Worrying about sleep creates physiological arousal that interferes with sleep. This can lead to conditioned arousal, where the bed becomes a cue for wakefulness.

- **Sleep effort is counterproductive:** Trying hard to sleep creates tension and alertness that prevent sleep from occurring.

Chapter 3: Assessing Your Sleep and Setting Goals

Now that you understand the basics of sleep science and the factors that contribute to insomnia, it's time to take a closer look at your own sleep patterns. Before we can start implementing changes, we need a clear picture of where you are starting from. This is the assessment phase.

Think of it like planning a road trip. You need to know your starting point before you can map out the route to your destination. This chapter will guide you through assessing the severity of your insomnia, identifying unhelpful beliefs, and, most importantly, starting a daily sleep diary.

Accurate self-assessment is crucial for the success of CBT-I. It allows us to tailor the strategies to your specific needs and track your progress. We will also talk about setting realistic goals.

Self-Assessment: The Insomnia Severity Index (ISI)

The first step is to measure the severity of your insomnia. The Insomnia Severity Index (ISI) is a brief, widely used questionnaire designed to measure your perception of your insomnia and its impact on your daily life (Bastien et al., 2001).

The ISI consists of seven questions that ask you to rate the severity of your sleep problems over the past two weeks. The questions cover:

1. Difficulty falling asleep.

2. Difficulty staying asleep.

3. Waking up too early.

4. Satisfaction with your current sleep pattern.

5. How noticeable your sleep problems are to others.

6. How worried or distressed you are about your sleep problems.

7. How much your sleep problems interfere with your daily functioning (e.g., mood, energy, concentration).

Each question is rated on a scale of 0 to 4. The total score ranges from 0 to 28. Higher scores indicate more severe insomnia.

Interpreting the ISI Score:

- **0-7:** No clinically significant insomnia.

- **8-14:** Subthreshold insomnia (mild insomnia).

- **15-21:** Clinical insomnia (moderate severity).

- **22-28:** Clinical insomnia (severe severity).

Completing the ISI now will give you a baseline measure. You will complete it again throughout the program to track your progress. It can be very motivating to see your score decrease over time.

(Workbook Activity: In a physical workbook, the full ISI questionnaire would be provided here.)

It's important to remember that the ISI measures your subjective experience. Your perception of your sleep is just as important as the objective measures (like how long you actually slept). Insomnia is defined not just by sleep difficulty, but also by the distress it causes.

Identifying unhelpful beliefs: The Dysfunctional Beliefs and Attitudes about Sleep (DBAS) Scale

As we discussed, unhelpful thoughts and beliefs about sleep play a significant role in perpetuating insomnia. Worrying about sleep loss, holding unrealistic expectations, and misunderstanding the causes of insomnia can all contribute to anxiety that interferes with sleep.

The Dysfunctional Beliefs and Attitudes about Sleep (DBAS) Scale is a questionnaire designed to identify and measure these unhelpful beliefs (Morin et al., 1993).

The DBAS Scale typically includes statements like:

- "I need 8 hours of sleep to feel refreshed and function well during the day."

- "When I have a bad night's sleep, I know it will interfere with my daily activities the next day."

- "I am worried that I may lose control over my abilities to sleep."

- "After a poor night's sleep, I should cancel my appointments or stay home from work."

- "Medication is probably the only solution to sleeplessness."

You rate how strongly you agree or disagree with each statement. Higher scores indicate a greater number of dysfunctional beliefs.

Why the DBAS is Important:

Identifying your specific unhelpful beliefs is the first step toward changing them. Once you know what thoughts are fueling your anxiety, you can start to challenge and replace them with more balanced perspectives. This is the core of the cognitive restructuring component of CBT-I, which we will cover later.

For now, completing the DBAS will help you become more aware of your attitudes toward sleep. You might be surprised by how many of these beliefs you hold without even realizing it.

(Workbook Activity: A selection of key items from the DBAS-16 scale would be provided here.)

Let's look at a case example of how dysfunctional beliefs can impact sleep.

Case Example: James

James had insomnia for years. He strongly believed that if he didn't get at least 7 hours of sleep, he would be unable to concentrate and might even get sick. Whenever he had a bad night, he would spend the next day feeling anxious and hyper-focused on his fatigue. He attributed every mistake at work to his lack of sleep. This belief created enormous pressure to sleep, which, predictably, made it harder for him to fall asleep. By challenging this belief, James was able to reduce his anxiety. He learned that while he might not feel his best after a bad night, he could still function reasonably well.

The crucial role of the Sleep Diary

While questionnaires provide valuable information, the single most important assessment tool in CBT-I is the *Sleep Diary*.

A Sleep Diary is a daily log where you record detailed information about your sleep patterns and habits. You complete it every morning shortly after waking up.

Why is the Sleep Diary so important?

1. It provides accurate information about your sleep:

When you have insomnia, your perception of your sleep can be distorted. You might overestimate how long it takes you to fall asleep and underestimate how much you actually slept. This is called sleep state misperception. The Sleep Diary helps provide a more objective picture.

2. It identifies patterns and factors affecting your sleep:

By tracking your daily habits (like caffeine intake, exercise, and bedtime routines) alongside your sleep patterns, the Sleep Diary can help you identify factors that might be interfering with your sleep.

3. It is used to tailor CBT-I strategies:

The information from your Sleep Diary is used to calculate your personalized sleep schedule for techniques like Sleep Restriction

Therapy. Without accurate data, these strategies cannot be implemented effectively.

4. It helps track your progress:

The Sleep Diary allows you to monitor changes over time. You can see improvements in how long it takes you to fall asleep and the overall quality of your sleep.

5. It increases awareness and accountability:

The simple act of tracking your sleep increases your awareness of your habits and motivates you to make changes.

Commitment to the Sleep Diary:

Keeping a daily Sleep Diary is a core commitment of the CBT-I program. It is essential that you complete it every day, as accurately and honestly as possible. It only takes a few minutes each morning.

You should continue keeping the Sleep Diary throughout the entire program (6-8 weeks).

How to complete a Sleep Diary accurately (instructions and examples)

A typical Sleep Diary includes the following information:

1. **Date and Day of the Week.**

2. **What time did you get into bed?**

3. **What time did you turn off the lights (try to sleep)?**

4. **How long did it take you to fall asleep?** (Your *sleep latency*).

5. **How many times did you wake up during the night?**

6. **How long were you awake during the night (total time)?** (Your *wake time after sleep onset* or WASO).

7. **What time did you wake up in the morning (final awakening)?**

8. **What time did you get out of bed in the morning?**

9. **How long did you sleep in total?** (Your *total sleep time* or TST).

10. **How would you rate the quality of your sleep?** (Usually on a scale of 1-5, from very poor to very good).

11. **Did you take any medications or substances (caffeine, alcohol, sleep aids)?**

12. **Comments/Notes:** (Anything unusual, such as stress or illness).

(Workbook Activity: A sample blank Sleep Diary template and a completed example would be provided here.)

Tips for Accurate Completion:

Completing the Sleep Diary accurately can be challenging, especially when you are tired. Here are some tips:

1. Complete it in the morning:

Fill it out shortly after waking up, while the information is fresh. Don't wait until later in the day.

2. Estimate, don't obsess:

Be accurate, but don't obsess over getting the exact times down to the minute. Your best estimate is good enough. The goal is to capture the overall pattern.

3. Do NOT watch the clock:

This is perhaps the most important rule. Watching the clock during the night increases anxiety and frustration, making it harder to sleep.

If you have a clock in your bedroom, turn it away from you. If you use your phone as an alarm, place it face down or across the room.

If you wake up during the night, do not check the time. Simply estimate how long you were awake based on your subjective feeling. For example, "I think I was awake for about 30 minutes."

4. Be honest:

Be honest about your habits, like caffeine intake or alcohol consumption. Remember, you are doing this for yourself. Accurate data is essential.

5. Don't worry about "bad data":

There will be nights when your sleep is particularly bad, or when you have difficulty estimating your sleep times. That's okay. Don't get discouraged. The important thing is the overall trend over time.

The Baseline Week:

Before starting the behavioral strategies of CBT-I, you need to complete a baseline week of Sleep Diaries. This means tracking your sleep for 7 consecutive days without making any changes to your habits or routines. This baseline data provides a clear picture of your current sleep patterns.

Calculating Sleep Efficiency (SE)

Once you have completed a week of Sleep Diaries, you can calculate an important measure called *Sleep Efficiency (SE)*.

Sleep Efficiency is the percentage of time spent asleep while in bed. It is a measure of the quality and consolidation of your sleep. A high SE means you are spending most of your time in bed actually sleeping. A low SE means you are spending a significant amount of time in bed awake.

The Formula for Sleep Efficiency:

Sleep Efficiency (SE) = (Total Sleep Time (TST) / Time In Bed (TIB)) x 100

- **Total Sleep Time (TST):** The total time you actually slept (from your Sleep Diary).

- **Time In Bed (TIB):** The total time you spent in bed, from the time you turned off the lights to the time you got out of bed (from your Sleep Diary).

Example Calculation:

Let's say your Sleep Diary shows the following:

- Turned off lights: 11:00 PM

- Fell asleep: 11:45 PM

- Woke up during the night: 1 hour (60 minutes)

- Final awakening: 6:30 AM

- Got out of bed: 7:00 AM

1. **Calculate Total Sleep Time (TST):**

   o Time from lights out to final awakening: 11:00 PM to 6:30 AM = 7 hours 30 minutes (450 minutes).

   o Time spent awake: 45 minutes (falling asleep) + 60 minutes (during the night) = 105 minutes.

   o TST = 450 minutes - 105 minutes = 345 minutes (5 hours 45 minutes).

2. **Calculate Time In Bed (TIB):**

   o Time from lights out to getting out of bed: 11:00 PM to 7:00 AM = 8 hours (480 minutes).

3. **Calculate Sleep Efficiency (SE):**

   o SE = (345 minutes / 480 minutes) x 100 = 71.9%

Interpreting Sleep Efficiency:

- **85% or higher:** Normal Sleep Efficiency. Good sleepers typically have an SE of 85% or higher.

- **80% - 84%:** Borderline Sleep Efficiency.

- **Less than 80%:** Low Sleep Efficiency. People with insomnia often have an SE of 70% or lower.

Calculating Weekly Average Sleep Efficiency:

To get a reliable measure, calculate your average Sleep Efficiency over the course of a week.

1. Calculate your TST and TIB for each night.

2. Add up the total TST for the week.

3. Add up the total TIB for the week.

4. Calculate the weekly average SE: (Total Weekly TST / Total Weekly TIB) x 100.

(Workbook Activity: A worksheet would be provided here to guide the reader through calculating their weekly average Sleep Efficiency.)

The Importance of Sleep Efficiency:

Sleep Efficiency is a key metric in CBT-I. The goal of the program is to increase your SE, leading to more consolidated sleep. The behavioral strategies we will introduce are designed specifically to improve Sleep Efficiency by reducing the time spent in bed awake.

Setting SMART goals for sleep improvement

Now that you have a clearer understanding of your baseline sleep patterns, it's time to set goals. Setting clear, realistic goals will help you stay motivated and focused.

When setting goals, it's helpful to use the SMART criteria. SMART goals are:

- **Specific:** Clearly defined and focused.

- **Measurable:** You can track your progress.

- **Achievable:** Realistic and attainable.

- **Relevant:** Meaningful to you.

- **Time-bound:** Have a specific timeframe.

Setting Realistic Expectations:

Before setting your goals, remember the importance of realistic expectations. The goal is not perfect sleep every night. The goal is improvement.

Examples of SMART Sleep Goals:

Here are some examples of SMART goals:

- **Goal 1: Improve Sleep Onset:**

  - *Not SMART:* "I want to fall asleep faster."

  - *SMART:* "I want to reduce the average time it takes me to fall asleep to 30 minutes or less within 6 weeks."

- **Goal 2: Improve Sleep Efficiency:**

  - *Not SMART:* "I want to sleep better."

  - *SMART:* "I want to increase my average Sleep Efficiency to 85% or higher within 8 weeks."

- **Goal 3: Improve Daytime Functioning:**

  - *Not SMART:* "I want to feel less tired."

  - *SMART:* "I want to have enough energy to exercise for 30 minutes three times a week within 4 weeks."

Focus on Behaviors, Not Just Outcomes:

It's also important to set behavioral goals—specific actions you will take. Sleep outcomes are not entirely under your control, but your behaviors are.

Examples of behavioral goals:

- "I will wake up at 6:00 AM every day, including weekends, for the next 4 weeks."

- "I will get out of bed if I am awake for more than 20 minutes during the night."

- "I will practice a relaxation technique for 15 minutes every evening before bed."

- "I will complete my Sleep Diary every morning for the next 8 weeks."

(Workbook Activity: A worksheet would be provided here to guide the reader in setting their own SMART goals.)

By setting clear and realistic goals, you are creating a roadmap for your journey toward better sleep.

Activity: Complete your baseline week of Sleep Diaries

Your task for the next week is to complete your baseline week of Sleep Diaries. Starting tonight, track your sleep every day for 7 consecutive days.

Instructions for the Baseline Week:

1. **Do not change anything:** During this baseline week, do not try to change your sleep habits or routines. Continue with your usual lifestyle. The goal is to capture a representative picture of your current sleep patterns.

2. **Be accurate and consistent:** Complete the Sleep Diary every morning. Estimate your times as accurately as possible, without watching the clock during the night.

3. **Calculate your weekly averages:** At the end of the week, calculate your weekly average Total Sleep Time (TST), Time In Bed (TIB), and Sleep Efficiency (SE).

This baseline data is essential for the next phase of the program, where we will start implementing the behavioral strategies of CBT-I.

In the next chapter, we will introduce Stimulus Control Therapy, one of the most powerful techniques for breaking the association between the bed and wakefulness. But first, focus on collecting accurate baseline data. This is the foundation.

Assessing Your Sleep Summary

- **Assessment is key:** Understanding your baseline sleep patterns is crucial for tailoring the CBT-I program and tracking your progress.

- **Measure severity:** The Insomnia Severity Index (ISI) measures the severity of your insomnia and its impact on your daily life.

- **Identify beliefs:** The Dysfunctional Beliefs and Attitudes about Sleep (DBAS) Scale identifies unhelpful thoughts and beliefs that contribute to insomnia.

- **The Sleep Diary is essential:** A daily Sleep Diary provides accurate information about your sleep patterns, habits, and factors affecting your sleep.

- **Accurate completion:** Complete the Sleep Diary every morning, estimating times without watching the clock.

- **Calculate Sleep Efficiency (SE):** SE is the percentage of time spent asleep while in bed. It is a key measure of sleep quality.

- **Set SMART goals:** Set specific, measurable, achievable, relevant, and time-bound goals for sleep improvement.

- **Baseline week:** Complete a baseline week of Sleep Diaries without changing your habits to capture your current sleep patterns.

Chapter 4: Stimulus Control Therapy (SCT)

We've spent the first few chapters laying the groundwork. You understand how sleep works, what keeps insomnia going, and you've been tracking your sleep patterns. That's great. Knowledge is important. But here's the deal: knowledge alone won't fix your sleep. To see real change, you have to take action.

This chapter marks a turning point in the workbook. We are moving from the *why* to the *how*. We are starting the behavioral strategies of CBT-I. And these strategies? They are powerful.

We begin with Stimulus Control Therapy, or SCT. This is often the first intervention introduced because it directly addresses one of the core problems in chronic insomnia: the broken association between your bed and sleep. SCT was developed in the 1970s by Dr. Richard Bootzin (Bootzin, 1972). It remains one of the most effective behavioral treatments for insomnia.

The goal of SCT is simple: to retrain your brain to associate your bed with sleep, and only sleep. It's about strengthening the cue (the stimulus) for sleep.

The problem of conditioned arousal Why your bed might be a cue for wakefulness

To understand why Stimulus Control is so necessary, we need to talk about *conditioned arousal*.

You might remember learning about Pavlov's dogs in school. Ivan Pavlov, a Russian physiologist, conducted experiments where he would ring a bell every time he fed his dogs. The dogs naturally salivated when they saw the food. After a while, the dogs started to salivate just hearing the bell, even when no food was present. They had learned to associate the bell (a neutral stimulus) with food (a stimulus that naturally causes salivation). This is called *classical conditioning*.

Now, how does this relate to insomnia? Well, you might be accidentally training yourself to be awake in bed.

Think about what happens when you have insomnia. You get into bed. You can't sleep. You toss and turn. You worry. You check the clock. You feel frustrated, anxious, and alert. Your mind races. You might watch TV, scroll through your phone, or even work in bed, hoping to distract yourself until sleep arrives.

If this happens night after night, your brain starts to connect the dots. It learns to associate your bed (the stimulus) with wakefulness, frustration, and mental activity (the response). The bed stops being a cue for sleep and becomes a cue for arousal.

This is conditioned arousal.

It explains that frustrating feeling of being exhausted on the couch while watching TV, barely able to keep your eyes open, but as soon as you move to the bedroom and get into bed—BAM! You're wide awake. Your mind switches on. It's not that you aren't tired. It's that your brain has been conditioned to expect arousal when you are in bed.

Case Example: Chloe

Chloe had struggled with sleep maintenance insomnia for two years. She would fall asleep fine, but wake up around 1 AM and stay awake for hours. During these hours, she would lie in bed, ruminating about her finances. She would often grab her tablet and start budgeting or browsing online shopping sites, thinking it would tire her out. When she started CBT-I, she realized her bed had become her "worry center." She associated the darkness and quiet of her bedroom with anxiety and mental alertness. She needed to break this association.

The goal of Stimulus Control Therapy is to reverse this conditioning. We want to extinguish the association between the bed and wakefulness, and re-establish the association between the bed and sleep. We want your brain to see the bed and immediately think, "Time to sleep."

How do we do this? By following a set of specific rules designed to ensure that you spend as much time as possible in bed asleep, and as little time as possible in bed awake.

The core rules of Stimulus Control

Stimulus Control Therapy consists of five core instructions. These rules might seem simple, maybe even obvious. But implementing them consistently requires commitment. They can also feel counterintuitive at first. You might resist some of them. That's normal. But trust the process. These rules are based on solid behavioral science.

Here are the five rules of Stimulus Control:

1. The bed is for sleep and sex only.

2. Go to bed only when sleepy.

3. If you can't sleep (the 15-20 Minute Rule), get out of bed.

4. Maintain a consistent wake time, 7 days a week.

5. Avoid daytime napping.

Let's break down each rule and the reasoning behind it.

The bed is for sleep and sex only

This is the golden rule of Stimulus Control. Your bed should be reserved exclusively for sleep. The only exception is sexual activity.

What does this mean in practice?

- **No watching TV in bed.**

- **No reading in bed.** (This one is often debated, but for people with severe insomnia, even reading can reinforce the association between the bed and wakefulness. We recommend reading on the couch or a comfortable chair until you are sleepy.)

- **No eating in bed.**

- **No working, studying, or using laptops/tablets in bed.**

- **No worrying or planning in bed.** (Easier said than done, I know. But if you find yourself worrying, it's better to get out of bed.)

- **And crucially, no scrolling on your phone in bed.** The blue light emitted by phones and tablets can suppress the release of melatonin, the sleep hormone, making it harder to fall asleep (Chang et al., 2015).

Why is this so strict? Because every time you engage in activities other than sleep in your bed, you weaken the association between the bed and sleep. You are sending mixed signals to your brain. You are teaching it that the bed is a place for entertainment, work, or worry.

By limiting the activities in bed to sleep and sex, you strengthen the connection. The bed becomes a powerful cue for sleep.

Common Challenges:

- *"But I love reading in bed to relax!"* I get it. It's a cozy habit. But if you have chronic insomnia, this habit might be working against you. Try reading in a different comfortable spot. If your sleep improves significantly, you might be able to gradually reintroduce reading in bed later, but for now, it's best to avoid it.

- *"My bedroom is my only private space."* If you live in a small apartment or with roommates, this can be challenging. Try to create a designated area in your bedroom, separate from the bed, for waking activities. Even a small chair in the corner can work. The key is that the bed itself remains sacred.

Go to bed only when sleepy

This rule sounds simple, but it's often misunderstood. Many people with insomnia go to bed when they think they *should* sleep, or when they are tired, but not necessarily *sleepy*.

There is a big difference between being tired and being sleepy.

- *Tiredness* (or fatigue) is a feeling of low energy, exhaustion, or physical weariness. You might feel tired all day when you have insomnia.

- *Sleepiness* (or drowsiness) is the strong urge to fall asleep. It's the feeling of heavy eyelids, nodding off, and struggling to stay awake.

If you go to bed when you are tired but not sleepy, you will likely lie there awake. Your mind might be active, even if your body is fatigued. This increases the time spent in bed awake, reinforcing conditioned arousal.

How to know if you are sleepy:

Pay attention to the physical signs of sleepiness. Are your eyes drooping? Are you yawning repeatedly? Are you having trouble focusing? If you are sitting on the couch and feel like you could easily drift off, that's sleepiness.

Wait for sleepiness:

This means you might have to stay up later than you are used to. If your usual bedtime is 10 PM, but you don't feel sleepy until 11:30 PM, stay up until 11:30 PM. Engage in relaxing activities during this time—reading, listening to calming music, light stretching. Avoid stimulating activities like intense exercise, emotional conversations, or watching suspenseful TV shows.

The goal is to reduce *sleep onset latency*—the time it takes you to fall asleep once you get into bed. By waiting until you are truly sleepy, you increase the likelihood that you will fall asleep quickly. This strengthens the positive association between the bed and sleep.

Common Challenges:

- *"I never feel sleepy."* Some people with insomnia have difficulty recognizing the signs of sleepiness. They might feel "wired" or hyperaroused in the evening. If this is the case, focus on creating a relaxing wind-down routine and still delay your bedtime slightly. The strategies we will discuss in the next chapter (Sleep Restriction) will help increase your sleep drive, making sleepiness more apparent.

- *"What if I get a second wind?"* Sometimes, if you stay up late, you might feel a burst of energy. This is your circadian rhythm kicking in. If this happens, continue with relaxing activities and wait for the next wave of sleepiness.

The 15-20 Minute Rule (getting out of bed if unable to sleep)

This is the most important, and often the most challenging, rule of Stimulus Control.

If you get into bed and cannot fall asleep within approximately 15-20 minutes, or if you wake up during the night and cannot fall back asleep within 15-20 minutes, you must get out of bed.

Why? Because lying in bed awake, trying to force sleep, is the engine that drives conditioned arousal. The frustration and anxiety build, making sleep impossible. You are training your brain to associate the bed with struggle.

By getting out of bed, you break this cycle. You prevent the negative association from forming.

How to apply the 15-20 Minute Rule:

1. **Estimate the time:** Do not watch the clock. This is crucial. Clock-watching increases anxiety. Estimate how long you have been awake based on your subjective feeling. If you feel like it's been "too long" (around 15-20 minutes), or if you start to feel frustrated, get up.

2. **Go to another room:** If possible, go to a different room. If you must stay in the bedroom, sit in a comfortable chair.

3. **Do something relaxing and quiet:** Engage in a calm, low-stimulation activity. Read a book (something engaging but not too exciting), listen to a podcast or audiobook, knit, do a puzzle, or practice a relaxation technique. Keep the lights dim.

4. **Avoid stimulating activities:** Do not watch TV (unless it's very boring), do not use your phone or computer, do not do chores, and do not eat a large meal.

5. **Return to bed only when sleepy:** Stay out of bed until you feel sleepy again. Once you feel drowsy, return to bed.

6. **Repeat if necessary:** If you return to bed and still cannot sleep within 15-20 minutes, get up again. Repeat this process as many times as needed throughout the night.

Yes, you read that right. As many times as needed. You might have to get up multiple times during the night, especially in the beginning. This is the hard part. It requires discipline and persistence.

The Rationale:

The goal is not to make you sleep more immediately. In fact, you might sleep less in the short term. The goal is to retrain your brain. By consistently removing yourself from the bed when you are awake, you are teaching your brain that the bed is only for sleep.

Over time, you will find that you fall asleep faster and wake up less frequently. The conditioned arousal will fade.

Case Example: Mark's implementation

Mark struggled with waking up at 2 AM and staying awake for hours. He started implementing the 15-20 minute rule. When he woke up, instead of lying there frustrated, he went to the living room and read a history book with a dim light. Sometimes he would read for an hour before feeling sleepy again. The first few nights were tough. He felt more tired during the day. But after a week, he noticed something shift. When he returned to bed, he fell asleep faster. And sometimes, when he woke up, he was able to fall back asleep without getting up. The association between the bed and frustration was starting to break.

Common Challenges:

- *"It's too cold/uncomfortable to get out of bed."* Prepare in advance. Have a robe and slippers ready. Make sure the place where you will go (your "sleep escape pod") is comfortable.

- *"I don't want to disturb my partner."* This is a valid concern. Discuss the plan with your partner beforehand. Explain why you are doing this. Remember, your chronic insomnia is probably already disturbing your partner. This is a short-term disruption for a long-term solution.

- *"I'm too tired to get up."* You might feel fatigued, but if your mind is active and you are not falling asleep, you are not sleepy enough. Getting up is the necessary action.

Maintain a consistent wake time, 7 days a week

This rule is essential for regulating your internal biological clock—the circadian rhythm.

Wake up at the same time every morning, regardless of how much you slept the night before, and including weekends.

Why is this so important?

Your wake time is the anchor for your circadian rhythm. It signals to your brain when the day begins. When your wake time is consistent, your internal clock stabilizes. This helps regulate the timing of sleepiness and alertness.

If you sleep in late on weekends, or if your wake time varies from day to day, you confuse your internal clock. This is what we called *social jetlag*. It's like constantly shifting time zones. It makes it harder to fall asleep at a consistent time in the evening.

How to implement this rule:

1. **Choose a realistic wake time:** Select a wake time that you can maintain consistently, based on your work or family obligations.

2. **Set an alarm and stick to it:** When the alarm goes off, get out of bed immediately. Do not hit the snooze button.

3. **Get exposed to bright light:** As soon as you wake up, expose yourself to bright light. Open the curtains, turn on the lights, or go outside if possible. Light is the strongest cue for synchronizing your circadian rhythm.

The Benefit:

A consistent wake time also helps build up your *homeostatic sleep drive* (sleep pressure). If you wake up at the same time every day, your sleep drive starts building at the same time, ensuring you have enough pressure to fall asleep at night.

If you had a bad night and slept very little, it might be tempting to sleep in. Don't. Sticking to your wake time will increase your sleep drive for the following night, making it more likely that you will sleep better.

Common Challenges:

- *"But I need to catch up on sleep on weekends!"* This is a myth. Trying to catch up on sleep disrupts your rhythm and perpetuates insomnia. Consistency is key.

- *"It's so hard to wake up when I'm exhausted."* Yes, it is. This requires discipline. But remember the long-term goal.

Sticking to your wake time is one of the most powerful things you can do to improve your sleep.

Avoid daytime napping

The final rule of Stimulus Control is to avoid daytime naps.

Why? Because napping reduces your homeostatic sleep drive. Remember the analogy of the sleep pressure balloon? When you nap, you release some of the pressure. This makes it harder to fall asleep and stay asleep at night.

For people with insomnia, daytime napping can be a major perpetuating factor. It's a vicious cycle: you sleep poorly at night, so you nap during the day, which leads to poorer sleep at night.

How to implement this rule:

The best strategy is to avoid napping altogether. If you feel sleepy during the day, try to push through it. Engage in light physical activity, drink some water, or get some fresh air.

Exceptions:

- **Safety:** If you are so sleepy that it is unsafe to drive or operate machinery, a brief nap might be necessary.
- **Illness:** If you are sick, your body might need extra rest.

If you must nap:

If a nap is unavoidable, keep it short and early.

- **Short:** Limit the nap to 20-30 minutes. This prevents you from entering deep sleep, which can make you feel groggy (sleep inertia) and significantly reduce your sleep drive.
- **Early:** Nap early in the afternoon (before 2-3 PM). Napping late in the day has a stronger negative impact on nighttime sleep.

However, during the initial stages of CBT-I, especially when implementing Stimulus Control and Sleep Restriction (next chapter), it is strongly recommended to avoid all naps if possible. We want to maximize your sleep drive for nighttime sleep.

Workbook Activity: Stimulus Control Implementation Plan and troubleshooting

Now it's time to put these rules into practice. Implementing Stimulus Control requires planning and preparation.

(In a physical workbook, this section would include worksheets to help the reader develop their plan.)

1. Set your Consistent Wake Time (CWT):

What time will you wake up every morning, 7 days a week? Choose a time that is realistic and sustainable.

My CWT is: _____

2. Prepare your sleep environment:

How will you ensure your bed is only for sleep?

- Remove the TV from the bedroom?

- Move your phone charger away from the bed?

- Create a designated space for reading or other activities outside the bed?

- Remove or cover all visible clocks from the bedroom.

3. Plan your wind-down routine:

What relaxing activities will you do in the evening while waiting for sleepiness?

- Reading a book on the couch?

- Listening to calming music?

- Practicing relaxation techniques (we will cover these later)?

4. Prepare for the 15-20 Minute Rule (Your "Sleep Escape Pod"):

What will you do when you get out of bed during the night? Prepare this space in advance.

- Where will you go? (Living room, kitchen, a chair in the bedroom?)
- What activity will you do? (Have a book ready, a podcast queued up?)
- How will you stay comfortable? (Robe, slippers, blanket?)

5. Plan for avoiding naps:

How will you manage daytime sleepiness without napping?

- Going for a short walk?
- Engaging in a stimulating conversation?
- Drinking cold water?

Troubleshooting Common Problems:

Anticipate challenges and develop strategies to overcome them.

Challenge: Resistance to getting out of bed.

Strategy: Remind yourself of the rationale. Lying in bed awake fuels insomnia. Getting up is the solution. Commit to trying it consistently for at least two weeks.

Challenge: Difficulty recognizing sleepiness.

Strategy: Pay close attention to the physical signs of drowsiness (heavy eyelids, nodding off). If you are unsure, err on the side of staying up later.

Challenge: Clock-watching.

Strategy: Remove or cover all clocks. Trust your internal estimation of time. If you feel frustrated, get up.

Challenge: Fear of increased daytime sleepiness.

Strategy: Acknowledge that you might feel more tired in the short term. This is a normal part of the process. The increased sleepiness will help improve your sleep in the long run. Prioritize safety (avoid driving drowsy).

Consistency is Key:

The effectiveness of Stimulus Control depends entirely on consistency. You cannot apply the rules selectively. You need to adhere to them every night, even when it's difficult.

It takes time to retrain your brain. Don't expect immediate results. It might take 2-3 weeks of consistent implementation to see significant improvements. But if you stick with it, Stimulus Control can dramatically improve the quality and consolidation of your sleep.

In the next chapter, we will introduce another powerful behavioral strategy: Sleep Restriction Therapy. This technique works hand-in-hand with Stimulus Control to increase your sleep drive and further consolidate your sleep.

Stimulus Control Guidelines

- **Conditioned arousal is the problem:** Insomnia is often maintained by the learned association between the bed and wakefulness, frustration, and anxiety.

- **SCT retrains the brain:** Stimulus Control Therapy aims to break this negative association and re-establish the bed as a strong cue for sleep.

- **Rule 1: Bed for sleep and sex only:** Remove all other activities (reading, TV, phone use, worrying) from the bed.

- **Rule 2: Go to bed only when sleepy:** Wait for signs of drowsiness (heavy eyelids, nodding off). Distinguish sleepiness from fatigue.

- **Rule 3: The 15-20 Minute Rule:** If you can't sleep, get out of bed. Do something relaxing in another room and return only when sleepy. Repeat as needed.

- **Rule 4: Consistent wake time:** Wake up at the same time every day, 7 days a week, regardless of how much you slept. This anchors your internal clock.

- **Rule 5: Avoid daytime napping:** Napping reduces sleep drive, making it harder to sleep at night.

- **Consistency is crucial:** Apply these rules strictly and consistently. Expect some short-term difficulty, but trust the long-term effectiveness.

Chapter 5: Sleep Restriction Therapy (SRT) and Sleep Compression

We've started the process of retraining your brain to associate the bed with sleep using Stimulus Control. Now, we are going to introduce the second major behavioral technique in CBT-I: Sleep Restriction Therapy (SRT).

If the name sounds intimidating, I understand. "Sleep Restriction" sounds like the last thing someone with insomnia wants. You want *more* sleep, not less, right?

But here's the thing: SRT is one of the most effective components of CBT-I (Spielman et al., 1987). It directly addresses a common problem that perpetuates insomnia: spending too much time in bed awake.

While Stimulus Control focuses on *what* you do in bed (strengthening the association with sleep), SRT focuses on *how much time* you spend in bed (increasing sleep drive and efficiency). These two techniques work together synergistically to consolidate your sleep.

This chapter will explain the rationale behind SRT, guide you step-by-step through the process of calculating and adjusting your personalized sleep schedule, and provide strategies for managing the challenges. We will also discuss a gentler alternative called Sleep Compression.

The rationale behind SRT: Matching time in bed with actual sleep time

Let's look at a typical pattern for someone with insomnia.

Suppose you believe you need 8 hours of sleep. You go to bed at 10 PM and get out of bed at 8 AM. That's 10 hours in bed. But you only actually sleep for 5 hours. The other 5 hours are spent tossing and turning, trying to fall asleep, or lying awake in the middle of the night.

What does this pattern lead to?

1. Low Sleep Efficiency:

In this example, your Sleep Efficiency (time asleep / time in bed) is only 50% (5 hours / 10 hours). Remember, good sleepers typically have a Sleep Efficiency of 85% or higher. Low Sleep Efficiency means your sleep is fragmented and shallow.

2. Weakened Sleep Drive:

Spending excessive time in bed, even if you are awake, can weaken your homeostatic sleep drive. Your body adapts to the extended opportunity for sleep by spreading the sleep out thinly. It doesn't build up enough pressure for deep, consolidated sleep.

3. Increased Conditioned Arousal:

As we discussed in the last chapter, spending long periods in bed awake increases frustration and anxiety, strengthening the association between the bed and wakefulness.

The Goal of Sleep Restriction Therapy:

The core principle of SRT is to match the amount of time you spend in bed (your *sleep window*) with the amount of time you are currently sleeping.

By restricting the time allowed in bed, SRT achieves several things:

- **It increases Sleep Drive:** Limiting the opportunity for sleep leads to a mild state of sleep deprivation. This builds up a stronger homeostatic sleep drive. When you go to bed, you are more likely to fall asleep quickly and stay asleep.

- **It improves Sleep Efficiency:** By reducing the time spent in bed awake, your Sleep Efficiency automatically increases.

- **It consolidates Sleep:** The increased sleep drive leads to deeper, more consolidated sleep, with fewer awakenings.

- **It reduces Sleep Anxiety:** When you start falling asleep faster and sleeping more soundly, your anxiety about sleep decreases.

The Process:

SRT is a gradual process. You start by restricting your time in bed to match your current average sleep duration. This creates a tight sleep window. Then, as your sleep improves (as measured by your Sleep Efficiency), you gradually expand the sleep window, allowing for more time in bed.

It sounds counterintuitive, but by temporarily reducing the time you spend in bed, you ultimately increase the quality and duration of your sleep.

A Word of Caution:

SRT leads to increased daytime sleepiness, especially in the beginning. This is a necessary part of the process. However, it's crucial to prioritize safety.

- **Do not drive or operate heavy machinery when drowsy.** If you feel excessively sleepy, take precautions. Arrange alternative transportation if needed.

- **Consult your doctor:** If you have certain medical conditions, such as bipolar disorder (as SRT can trigger mania), untreated sleep apnea, or a history of seizures, SRT might need to be modified or avoided (Perlis et al., 2019). Consult with your healthcare provider before starting SRT if you have any concerns.

Step-by-step guide to calculating your personalized sleep window

The first step in implementing SRT is to calculate your personalized sleep window. This is the specific timeframe during which you are allowed to be in bed.

You will use the data from your baseline week of Sleep Diaries to determine this window.

Here is the step-by-step process:

Step 1: Calculate your Average Total Sleep Time (TST)

Look at your baseline week Sleep Diary. Calculate the Total Sleep Time (TST) for each night (the actual time you slept). Then, calculate the weekly average TST.

Example:

- Monday: 5h 30m (330 min)
- Tuesday: 6h 0m (360 min)
- Wednesday: 5h 0m (300 min)
- Thursday: 6h 30m (390 min)
- Friday: 5h 30m (330 min)
- Saturday: 6h 0m (360 min)
- Sunday: 5h 0m (300 min)

Total TST = 2370 minutes

Average TST = 2370 minutes / 7 days = 338.6 minutes (approx. 5 hours 40 minutes)

Step 2: Determine your Sleep Window Duration

Your initial sleep window will be equal to your Average Total Sleep Time (TST).

Important Rule: The Minimum Sleep Window

The sleep window should never be less than 5 hours, even if your Average TST is lower. This is for safety reasons, to ensure you get a minimum amount of sleep.

Example (continued):

Initial Sleep Window Duration = 5 hours 40 minutes.

Step 3: Establish your Sleep Window Schedule

Now you need to decide when your sleep window will occur. This is based on your Consistent Wake Time (CWT), which you established in the last chapter.

1. Start with your CWT: This is the time you must get out of bed every morning.

Example: CWT = 6:30 AM.

2. Calculate your Prescribed Bedtime: Count backward from your CWT by the duration of your sleep window.

Example: 6:30 AM minus 5 hours 40 minutes = 12:50 AM.

Your Prescribed Sleep Window is from 12:50 AM to 6:30 AM.

Step 4: Implement the Sleep Window

For the next week, you must adhere strictly to this sleep window.

- **Do not go to bed before your prescribed bedtime (12:50 AM).** Even if you feel sleepy earlier, you must stay up.

- **Get out of bed at your Consistent Wake Time (6:30 AM).** Even if you slept poorly and want to sleep longer, you must get up.

Staying up late:

This is often the most challenging part of SRT. You need to stay awake until your prescribed bedtime.

Plan activities to keep yourself occupied during this time. In the beginning, when your sleep drive is increasing, you might feel very sleepy in the evening.

- **Early evening:** Engage in more active tasks (chores, light exercise, socializing).

- **Late evening (closer to bedtime):** Switch to relaxing activities (reading, listening to music).

If you find yourself struggling to stay awake, get up and move around. Splash cold water on your face.

Case Example: David's SRT Calculation

David completed his baseline week Sleep Diary. His Average TST was 5 hours 15 minutes. He decided on a Consistent Wake Time of 7:00 AM.

His initial Sleep Window Duration was 5 hours 15 minutes.

His Prescribed Bedtime was 7:00 AM minus 5 hours 15 minutes = 1:45 AM.

David's Sleep Window was 1:45 AM to 7:00 AM.

David was used to going to bed at 11 PM. Staying up until 1:45 AM was a big adjustment. He planned his evenings to keep himself busy. He did laundry, prepared meals for the next day, and read books. The first few nights were difficult. He felt very sleepy around 10 PM. But he pushed through. When he finally went to bed at 1:45 AM, he fell asleep within minutes.

Continue tracking your sleep:

While implementing SRT, it is essential to continue completing your Sleep Diary every day. This data will be used to adjust your sleep window each week.

How to adjust your sleep window based on weekly Sleep Efficiency

SRT is not about permanently restricting your sleep. It's a dynamic process. You adjust your sleep window weekly based on your progress, as measured by your Sleep Efficiency (SE).

The goal is to gradually increase your sleep window as your sleep becomes more consolidated.

The Adjustment Process:

At the end of each week, calculate your weekly average Sleep Efficiency (SE).

Weekly Average SE = (Total Weekly TST / Total Weekly Time In Bed) x 100

(Note: Time In Bed should be equal to your prescribed sleep window duration if you adhered to the schedule.)

Based on your average SE, adjust your sleep window for the following week using these rules (the titration process):

Rule 1: If SE is 85% or higher (Good Sleep Efficiency): Increase the Sleep Window

If your sleep is consolidated (SE ≥ 85%), you can expand your sleep window by 15 minutes. This means moving your prescribed bedtime 15 minutes earlier.

Example:

If your Sleep Window is 12:50 AM - 6:30 AM, and your SE is 87%.

New Sleep Window: 12:35 AM - 6:30 AM.

Rule 2: If SE is between 80% and 84% (Borderline Sleep Efficiency): Keep the Sleep Window the Same

If your sleep efficiency is borderline, keep the same sleep window for another week. This gives your body more time to adjust and consolidate sleep at the current level.

Example:

If your Sleep Window is 12:50 AM - 6:30 AM, and your SE is 82%.

New Sleep Window: 12:50 AM - 6:30 AM.

Rule 3: If SE is less than 80% (Low Sleep Efficiency): Decrease the Sleep Window

If your sleep is still fragmented (SE < 80%), you need to tighten the sleep window further to increase sleep drive. Decrease the sleep window by 15 minutes. This means moving your prescribed bedtime 15 minutes later.

Example:

If your Sleep Window is 12:50 AM - 6:30 AM, and your SE is 75%.

New Sleep Window: 1:05 AM - 6:30 AM.

(Remember the minimum 5-hour sleep window rule. Never decrease it below 5 hours.)

Patience and Persistence:

SRT is a gradual process. It typically takes several weeks (6-8 weeks) to achieve the desired results.

There will be ups and downs. Some weeks you will make progress, and other weeks you might plateau or even have a setback. This is normal. The key is to stick with the process consistently.

Do not adjust your sleep window more frequently than once a week. Your body needs time to adapt to the changes.

Case Example: David's SRT Progress

Week 1: Sleep Window: 1:45 AM - 7:00 AM (5h 15m). Average SE: 88%.

Adjustment: Increase by 15 min.

Week 2: Sleep Window: 1:30 AM - 7:00 AM (5h 30m). Average SE: 86%.

Adjustment: Increase by 15 min.

Week 3: Sleep Window: 1:15 AM - 7:00 AM (5h 45m). Average SE: 83%.

Adjustment: Keep the same. (David had a stressful week, which affected his sleep.)

Week 4: Sleep Window: 1:15 AM - 7:00 AM (5h 45m). Average SE: 87%.

Adjustment: Increase by 15 min.

Week 5: Sleep Window: 1:00 AM - 7:00 AM (6h 0m).

Over five weeks, David increased his sleep duration from 5h 15m to 6h 0m, and his sleep quality improved significantly. He felt more refreshed during the day.

Strategies for managing daytime sleepiness during SRT

Let's be upfront: Sleep Restriction Therapy is challenging. By design, it causes mild sleep deprivation, which leads to increased daytime sleepiness. This is the hardest part of the program for many people.

However, this sleepiness is temporary and necessary. It is the driving force behind the consolidation of your sleep.

Here are some strategies to help you manage daytime sleepiness during SRT:

1. Prioritize Safety:

This is the most important point. Do not drive drowsy. If you feel excessively sleepy, avoid driving. Arrange for alternative transportation, work from home if possible, or take a brief safety nap if absolutely necessary (less than 20 minutes, early afternoon). Be cautious when operating machinery or performing tasks that require alertness.

2. Optimize your Environment:

- **Bright Light:** Expose yourself to bright light during the day, especially in the morning. This helps increase alertness by strengthening your circadian rhythm. Go outside for a walk if possible.

- **Cool Temperature:** Keep your environment slightly cool. Warm temperatures can increase drowsiness.

3. Behavioral Strategies:

- **Stay Active:** Engage in light physical activity throughout the day. Go for short walks, stretch at your desk. Exercise can increase alertness.

- **Stay Hydrated:** Drink plenty of water. Dehydration can worsen fatigue.

- **Engage in Stimulating Activities:** Engage in conversations, work on tasks that require focus (if possible), or listen to upbeat music.

4. Manage Caffeine Wisely:

Caffeine can be a useful tool to promote alertness during SRT. However, use it strategically.

- **Timing:** Consume caffeine only in the morning or early afternoon (before 2 PM). Avoid caffeine late in the day, as it can interfere with nighttime sleep.

- **Moderation:** Do not consume excessive amounts of caffeine.

5. Adjust your Schedule (if possible):

If possible, reduce your workload or social commitments during the initial stages of SRT. Avoid scheduling demanding tasks during times when you typically feel most sleepy (often the mid-afternoon dip).

6. Cognitive Strategies (Mindset):

- **Remind yourself of the rationale:** Remember why you are doing this. The temporary discomfort is an investment in your long-term sleep health.

- **Acknowledge the difficulty:** Be compassionate with yourself. It's okay to feel tired and irritable.

- **Focus on the progress:** Celebrate the small improvements in your sleep quality, even if the duration is still short.

When Sleepiness is Severe:

If you experience severe daytime sleepiness that interferes with your ability to function safely, you might need to modify the SRT protocol.

- **Increase the minimum sleep window:** If the 5-hour minimum is too restrictive, increase it to 5.5 or 6 hours.

- **Use Sleep Compression (see next section):** This gentler alternative might be more manageable.

Sleep Compression: A gentler alternative for gradual reduction of time in bed

Sleep Restriction Therapy is highly effective, but it can be demanding. The sudden reduction in time in bed and the resulting daytime sleepiness can be difficult for some people to tolerate.

If you find SRT too challenging, or if you are concerned about the safety implications of increased sleepiness (e.g., if you are a professional driver), *Sleep Compression* is a gentler alternative.

Sleep Compression works on the same principle as SRT—reducing the time spent in bed awake—but the process is more gradual.

The Process of Sleep Compression:

Instead of immediately reducing your time in bed to match your current sleep duration, you gradually reduce your time in bed over several weeks.

Here is the step-by-step process:

Step 1: Calculate your current Time In Bed (TIB) and Average Total Sleep Time (TST)

Use your baseline Sleep Diary data.

Example:

Average TST = 5 hours 30 minutes.

Average TIB = 8 hours 30 minutes (e.g., 10:00 PM to 6:30 AM).

Step 2: Gradually reduce your Time In Bed

Each week, reduce your Time In Bed by a small amount (e.g., 15-30 minutes). You can do this by either moving your bedtime later, or moving your wake time earlier (or a combination of both). However, maintaining a consistent wake time and moving the bedtime later is generally recommended to build sleep drive.

Example (reducing TIB by 30 minutes per week):

Week 1: TIB = 8 hours. Bedtime: 10:30 PM - 6:30 AM.

Week 2: TIB = 7 hours 30 minutes. Bedtime: 11:00 PM - 6:30 AM.

Week 3: TIB = 7 hours. Bedtime: 11:30 PM - 6:30 AM.

Week 4: TIB = 6 hours 30 minutes. Bedtime: 12:00 AM - 6:30 AM.

Step 3: Continue until TIB matches TST (or desired sleep duration)

Continue this gradual reduction until your Time In Bed is close to your Total Sleep Time, or until you reach a sleep duration that allows you to feel refreshed during the day and your Sleep Efficiency is high (85% or higher).

Advantages of Sleep Compression:

- **Gentler:** The gradual nature makes it easier to tolerate. Daytime sleepiness is less severe.

- **Safer:** Reduced risk of accidents due to extreme drowsiness.

- **Better adherence:** People are more likely to stick with the program if it is less demanding.

Disadvantages of Sleep Compression:

- **Slower:** It takes longer to see results compared to SRT.

- **Less potent:** The increase in sleep drive is less pronounced, so the consolidation of sleep might be less dramatic initially.

Choosing between SRT and Sleep Compression:

The choice depends on your individual circumstances, preferences, and the severity of your insomnia.

- **SRT might be better if:** You have severe insomnia, you want faster results, and you can tolerate increased daytime sleepiness safely.

- **Sleep Compression might be better if:** You have milder insomnia, you prefer a gradual approach, you are concerned about daytime sleepiness, or you have medical conditions that make SRT risky.

Both methods are effective if implemented consistently. The key is to choose the approach that you can stick with.

Workbook Activity: SRT Calculation and Adjustment Tracker

Now it's time to plan your implementation of SRT (or Sleep Compression).

(In a physical workbook, this section would include worksheets for calculation and tracking.)

Part 1: Calculation of Initial Sleep Window (if using SRT)

1. **Average Total Sleep Time (TST) (from baseline Sleep Diary):** _____ hours _____ minutes.

2. **Initial Sleep Window Duration (equal to Average TST, minimum 5 hours):** _____ hours _____ minutes.

3. **Consistent Wake Time (CWT):** _____.

4. **Prescribed Bedtime (CWT minus Sleep Window Duration):** _____.

5. **Initial Sleep Window:** _____ to _____.

Part 2: Planning for Implementation

1. **Start Date:** When will you begin implementing the new schedule?

2. **Strategies for staying up late:** What activities will you do in the evening?

3. **Strategies for managing daytime sleepiness:** How will you cope with increased drowsiness safely?

Part 3: Weekly Adjustment Tracker

Use this tracker to monitor your progress and adjust your sleep window weekly.

Week	Sleep Window (Bedtime - Wake Time)	Average TST	Average SE (%)	Adjustment (e.g., +15 min, -15 min, Same)	New Sleep Window
1					
2					
3					

Week	Sleep Window (Bedtime - Wake Time)	Average TST	Average SE (%)	Adjustment (e.g., +15 min, -15 min, Same)	New Sleep Window
4					
5					
6					

A Note on Combining SRT and Stimulus Control:

It is essential to implement SRT in conjunction with the Stimulus Control rules discussed in the previous chapter. They work together.

- Adhere to your prescribed sleep window (SRT).

- Go to bed only when sleepy (SC). (If you reach your prescribed bedtime but are not sleepy, stay up until you are sleepy. However, try to adhere to the bedtime as closely as possible).

- If you can't sleep, get out of bed (SC). (Even within the restricted sleep window, if you are awake for more than 15-20 minutes, get out of bed).

- Maintain your consistent wake time (SC/SRT).

- Avoid naps (SC/SRT).

Implementing these behavioral strategies requires significant effort, but the payoff is substantial. You are taking active steps to retrain your sleep system and reclaim your sleep.

In the next part of the workbook, we will shift our focus to the cognitive strategies—addressing the thoughts and beliefs that contribute to insomnia. But for the next few weeks, focus on consistently implementing these behavioral changes.

Sleep Restriction and Compression Review

- **SRT addresses excessive time in bed:** Sleep Restriction Therapy (SRT) matches the time allowed in bed with the actual time spent sleeping.

- **SRT increases sleep drive and efficiency:** By restricting the sleep window, SRT increases homeostatic sleep drive, leading to more consolidated sleep and improved Sleep Efficiency.

- **Calculate your sleep window:** Use your baseline Sleep Diary data to calculate your Average Total Sleep Time (TST). Your initial sleep window equals your Average TST (minimum 5 hours).

- **Establish a schedule:** Determine your prescribed bedtime based on your Consistent Wake Time (CWT). Adhere strictly to this schedule.

- **Adjust weekly based on SE:** Calculate your weekly average Sleep Efficiency (SE). Increase the sleep window by 15 minutes if SE ≥ 85%. Keep it the same if SE is 80-84%. Decrease by 15 minutes if SE < 80%.

- **Manage daytime sleepiness:** SRT causes temporary increased sleepiness. Prioritize safety (do not drive drowsy) and use strategies to manage drowsiness.

- **Sleep Compression is a gentler alternative:** Sleep Compression gradually reduces time in bed over several weeks. It is slower but easier to tolerate than SRT.

- **Consistency is key:** Both SRT and Sleep Compression require consistent implementation, in conjunction with Stimulus Control rules.

Chapter 6: Identifying Unhelpful Thoughts About Sleep

If you've been following the behavioral strategies in the last two chapters—Stimulus Control and Sleep Restriction—you might already be noticing some changes. Maybe you're falling asleep a bit faster, or your sleep feels slightly deeper. That's fantastic. Keep going.

But maybe you're finding that even when you follow the rules, your mind just won't shut off. You're lying in bed, you know you *should* be sleepy because your sleep drive is high, but your brain is buzzing with thoughts, worries, and frustration.

This is where the "C" in CBT-I comes in. Cognitive Behavioral Therapy addresses both behaviors (what you do) and cognitions (what you think). While the behavioral strategies help reset your body clock and increase your sleep drive, the cognitive strategies help calm your mind and change your relationship with sleep.

Insomnia isn't just a physical problem. It's deeply intertwined with your thoughts and emotions. This chapter is about understanding how your thinking patterns contribute to insomnia and learning how to identify the specific unhelpful thoughts that are keeping you awake.

The role of cognitive arousal in insomnia

When we talk about arousal in the context of sleep, we mean a state of alertness. To fall asleep, your body and mind need to wind down. Arousal needs to decrease.

Insomnia is often characterized by *hyperarousal*—a state of heightened physiological and cognitive activation (Riemann et al., 2010). It's like your "fight-or-flight" system is stuck in the "on" position.

Physiological arousal includes things like increased heart rate, muscle tension, and stress hormone levels. Cognitive arousal refers to the mental activity—the racing thoughts, worry, and mental alertness.

Cognitive arousal is a major factor in perpetuating insomnia. It creates a vicious cycle.

The Vicious Cycle of Cognitive Arousal:

1. **Trigger:** You have difficulty sleeping.

2. **Unhelpful Thoughts:** You start having thoughts like, "I'll never fall asleep," "Tomorrow is ruined," or "Why is this happening to me?"

3. **Emotional Response:** These thoughts trigger emotions like anxiety, frustration, and helplessness.

4. **Physiological Arousal:** These emotions activate the stress response, increasing physiological arousal.

5. **Sleep Interference:** The heightened state of arousal makes it even harder to sleep.

6. **More Unhelpful Thoughts:** The continued wakefulness leads to more worry and frustration, fueling the cycle.

The key insight from Cognitive Therapy, developed by Dr. Aaron Beck, is that it's not the situation itself that causes the emotional distress, but rather our interpretation of the situation—our thoughts (Beck, 1976).

If you view being awake at night as a catastrophe, you will feel anxious and aroused. If you view it as a temporary inconvenience, you might feel annoyed, but the level of arousal will be much lower, making it easier to eventually fall asleep.

The Content of Cognitive Arousal:

What are people thinking about when they are lying awake? The content can vary.

1. Worry about Sleep (Sleep Anxiety):

This is the most common type of cognitive arousal in insomnia. It involves worrying about the inability to sleep and the consequences of sleep loss.

- "If I don't get 7 hours, I won't be able to cope."
- "I must fall asleep now."
- "My insomnia is damaging my health."

This type of worry creates *sleep performance anxiety*. You feel pressure to perform (to sleep), and this pressure itself keeps you awake.

2. Worry about Daytime Consequences:

This involves worrying about how the lack of sleep will affect your functioning the next day.

- "I have an important meeting tomorrow; I'll mess it up if I don't sleep."
- "I'll be too tired to take care of my kids."
- "I'll feel miserable all day."

3. General Worry and Rumination:

Sometimes, the content is not directly related to sleep. You might find yourself worrying about work, finances, relationships, health, or reviewing past events (rumination). The quiet and darkness of the night can provide an opportunity for these thoughts to surface, especially if you avoid them during the day.

4. Problem-Solving and Planning:

Your mind might be busy trying to solve problems or plan for the future. This mental activity keeps you alert.

The Impact of Unhelpful Beliefs:

Underlying these immediate worries are often deeply held beliefs about sleep. Dr. Charles Morin identified that people with insomnia tend to hold "dysfunctional beliefs and attitudes about sleep" (Morin, 1993). We touched on this when discussing the DBAS scale in Chapter 3.

These beliefs can include:

- Unrealistic expectations about how much sleep is needed.

- Misconceptions about the causes of insomnia.

- Exaggerated beliefs about the consequences of sleep loss.

- A sense of helplessness about the ability to control sleep.

These beliefs fuel the cognitive arousal. If you believe that a single bad night of sleep is catastrophic, you will naturally react with intense anxiety.

The Goal of Cognitive Therapy:

The goal of the cognitive component of CBT-I is to reduce cognitive arousal by helping you identify and change these unhelpful thoughts and beliefs. We are not trying to eliminate all thoughts. That's impossible. We are trying to change your relationship with your thoughts, making them less distressing and less disruptive to sleep.

It's about shifting from a mindset of struggle and catastrophe to a mindset of acceptance and realistic appraisal.

Common cognitive distortions related to sleep

When we are anxious or stressed, our thinking can become distorted. We tend to see the world through a negative lens. These systematic errors in thinking are called *cognitive distortions*.

Cognitive distortions are like filters that twist reality. They lead to inaccurate conclusions and increased distress. Recognizing these distortions is the first step toward challenging them.

Here are some common cognitive distortions related to sleep (Morin & Espie, 2012):

1. Catastrophizing:

This involves exaggerating the negative consequences of a situation and assuming the worst-case scenario will happen. It's turning a molehill into a mountain.

In insomnia, catastrophizing often involves exaggerating the impact of a bad night's sleep.

Examples:

- "If I don't sleep well tonight, I will bomb my presentation tomorrow and lose my job."

- "My insomnia is going to cause a serious illness."

- "I will never have a normal life if I can't fix my sleep."

Catastrophizing creates intense anxiety and arousal.

2. All-or-Nothing Thinking (Black-and-White Thinking):

This involves seeing things in extreme categories, with no middle ground. Either you are a good sleeper or a terrible sleeper. Either you get 8 hours or your night is ruined.

Examples:

- "If I don't get 8 hours of sleep, I might as well not have slept at all."

- "I woke up in the middle of the night, so now the whole night is wasted."

- "If I can't function perfectly, I am useless."

This type of thinking ignores the reality that sleep quality and daytime functioning exist on a spectrum.

3. Overgeneralization:

This involves drawing a broad conclusion based on a single event. You take one negative experience and assume it will happen repeatedly.

Examples:

- "I had a bad night last night; I know I won't sleep well for the rest of the week."

- "CBT-I isn't working because I had a rough night."

- "I am just a bad sleeper."

Overgeneralization leads to feelings of helplessness and hopelessness.

4. Filtering (Selective Attention):

This involves focusing exclusively on the negative aspects of a situation and ignoring the positive ones.

In insomnia, this often involves focusing on the time spent awake and ignoring the time spent asleep. Or focusing on the feelings of fatigue during the day and ignoring the moments of alertness.

Examples:

- Lying awake for 30 minutes and concluding, "I didn't sleep at all," even if you slept for 6 hours.

- Attributing every mistake during the day to lack of sleep, while ignoring the things you accomplished.

Filtering reinforces the negative perception of your sleep.

5. Jumping to Conclusions (Mind Reading and Fortune Telling):

This involves making assumptions without evidence.

Fortune Telling: Predicting a negative outcome.

- "I know I won't be able to fall asleep tonight." (This can become a self-fulfilling prophecy).

Mind Reading: Assuming you know what others are thinking.

- "My partner is annoyed with me because I was tossing and turning."

6. Should Statements:

This involves having rigid rules about how you or others should behave. These "shoulds," "musts," and "oughts" create pressure and anxiety.

Examples:

- "I should be able to fall asleep within 10 minutes."

- "I must get enough sleep tonight."

- "I shouldn't feel tired during the day."

These unrealistic expectations lead to frustration when reality doesn't match up.

7. Misattribution:

This involves incorrectly assigning the cause of an event. In insomnia, this often involves attributing all daytime problems to lack of sleep, while ignoring other potential factors.

Examples:

- Feeling irritable and assuming it's solely due to lack of sleep, when it might also be related to stress at work or dehydration.

- Having difficulty concentrating and attributing it entirely to insomnia, while ignoring the impact of multitasking or distractions.

Misattribution increases the perceived impact of insomnia, fueling anxiety.

Case Example: Sarah's Cognitive Distortions

Sarah often woke up at 3 AM. Her mind would immediately start racing.

Thought 1: "Oh no, here we go again. I'll be awake for hours." (Overgeneralization and Fortune Telling).

Thought 2: "If I don't get back to sleep soon, I won't be able to handle my stressful job tomorrow. I might even get fired." (Catastrophizing).

Thought 3: "I should be able to sleep like a normal person. Why is my body failing me?" (Should Statement).

Thought 4: The next day, she felt tired and made a small mistake at work. She thought, "See? My insomnia is ruining my career." (Misattribution and Filtering).

These distorted thoughts created intense anxiety that kept Sarah awake. By learning to recognize these patterns, she could start to challenge them.

Recognizing your Automatic Negative Thoughts (ANTs) about sleep

The thoughts that pop into your head when you can't sleep are often *Automatic Negative Thoughts (ANTs)*. They are reflexive, rapid, and seem plausible, even if they are inaccurate.

They happen so quickly that you might not even notice them. You might just notice the feeling of anxiety or frustration that follows.

The goal of this section is to help you become more aware of your ANTs. You need to catch them before you can change them.

How to Identify Your ANTs:

1. Pay Attention to Your Emotions:

The first clue that you are having ANTs is a shift in your emotional state. When you are lying in bed and suddenly feel a wave of anxiety, frustration, or anger, ask yourself:

"What was going through my mind just before I felt this way?"

2. Identify Common Themes:

Look for patterns in your thoughts. Do you tend to worry about the impact on your health? Your performance at work? The loss of control?

3. Look for Cognitive Distortions:

Review the list of cognitive distortions above. Do you recognize any of these patterns in your thinking?

4. Complete a Thought Record:

The most effective way to identify ANTs is to use a Thought Record. This is a structured tool that helps you capture and analyze your thoughts. We will introduce the Thought Record in the next section.

Examples of Common ANTs related to sleep:

Here are some examples of common ANTs that people with insomnia experience. See if any of these resonate with you.

At Bedtime (Difficulty Falling Asleep):

- "I'll never fall asleep."
- "I'm trying so hard, why isn't it working?"
- "Everyone else is asleep; what's wrong with me?"
- "I need to clear my mind."
- "If I don't fall asleep in the next 10 minutes, I'm doomed."

During the Night (Difficulty Staying Asleep):

- "Oh no, I'm awake again."
- "I must get back to sleep immediately."
- "This is unbearable."

- "I wonder what time it is." (The urge to check the clock is often driven by anxiety).

- "I'll feel terrible in the morning."

During the Day (After a Bad Night):

- "I can't function today."

- "I look terrible."

- "I need to cancel my plans."

- "My day is ruined."

- "I need a nap." (The urge to nap can be driven by the belief that you cannot function without it).

The Importance of Recognizing ANTs:

Identifying your ANTs is a crucial skill. It allows you to create distance between yourself and your thoughts. You start to realize that **thoughts are not facts**. They are interpretations of reality, and they can be biased or inaccurate.

When you recognize an ANT, you can start to question its validity. Is this thought helpful? Is it accurate? What is the evidence for it?

This process of questioning and challenging your thoughts is called *Cognitive Restructuring*, which we will cover in the next chapter. But first, you need to practice catching those ANTs.

Workbook Activity: Sleep-Related Thought Record

The Thought Record is a powerful tool for identifying and analyzing your Automatic Negative Thoughts (ANTs). It helps you slow down your thinking process and examine the connection between your thoughts, emotions, and behaviors.

For the next week, use the Sleep-Related Thought Record whenever you experience difficulty sleeping or distress related to your sleep.

You can complete it during the night (if you are out of bed as part of Stimulus Control) or the next morning.

(In a physical workbook, a blank Thought Record template would be provided here. Here is a description of the columns):

Column 1: Situation/Trigger

Describe the situation or trigger that led to the distress. Be objective and specific.

Examples:

- "Woke up in the middle of the night and couldn't fall back asleep."

- "Lying in bed at the start of the night, mind racing."

- "Felt tired during the day after a bad night's sleep."

Column 2: Automatic Negative Thoughts (ANTs)

Write down the exact thoughts that went through your mind. What were you telling yourself?

Rate the intensity of your belief in each thought (0-100%).

Examples:

- "I'll never fall asleep." (90%)

- "Tomorrow will be ruined." (80%)

- "This is ruining my health." (70%)

Column 3: Emotions/Feelings

Write down the emotions you felt. (e.g., anxious, frustrated, angry, helpless, sad).

Rate the intensity of each emotion (0-100%).

Examples:

- Anxious (80%)

- Frustrated (90%)

- Helpless (70%)

Column 4: Cognitive Distortions

Identify the cognitive distortions present in your ANTs. (Refer to the list earlier in this chapter).

Examples:

- Catastrophizing

- Fortune Telling

- Overgeneralization

Example of a Completed Thought Record:

- **Situation/Trigger:** Woke up at 3 AM and felt wide awake.

- **Automatic Negative Thoughts (with belief %):**

  1. "Oh no, not again. I'm going to be awake for hours." (90%)
  2. "If I don't get enough sleep, I'll mess up my meeting tomorrow." (85%)
  3. "I can't stand this anymore." (95%)

- **Emotions/Feelings (with intensity %):**

  - Anxious (85%)
  - Frustrated (90%)
  - Desperate (80%)

- **Cognitive Distortions:**

  - Fortune-telling, Overgeneralization
  - Catastrophizing
  - Filtering (focusing only on negatives)

84

- **Evidence For the Thoughts:**

  - I sometimes do feel tired the next day after poor sleep.
  - My focus and patience can drop when I don't rest.

- **Evidence Against the Thoughts:**

  - I've had poor nights of sleep before and still got through important days.
  - Even when tired, I can perform well enough by pacing myself.
  - Worrying in the middle of the night makes it harder to fall back asleep.

- **Balanced Thought:**

"I can't predict how long I'll be awake. Even if I stay up, I've coped with tiredness before. Tomorrow I can prioritize important tasks, take breaks, and still manage my meeting. Right now, my job is to focus on resting, not panicking."

The Purpose of the Thought Record (at this stage):

At this stage, the goal is simply to identify the thoughts and recognize the patterns. We are not trying to change the thoughts yet. That comes next.

By practicing the Thought Record, you will become more aware of your cognitive arousal and the specific thoughts that fuel it. This awareness is the foundation for cognitive change.

Key Insights on Sleep Thoughts

- **Cognitive arousal fuels insomnia:** Racing thoughts, worry, and mental alertness (cognitive arousal) interfere with sleep and create a vicious cycle of anxiety and wakefulness.

- **Unhelpful beliefs underlie worry:** Dysfunctional beliefs about sleep (e.g., unrealistic expectations, exaggerated consequences) fuel cognitive arousal.

- **Cognitive distortions twist reality:** When anxious, our thinking can become distorted. Common distortions include catastrophizing, all-or-nothing thinking, overgeneralization, and filtering.

- **ANTs are reflexive and rapid:** Automatic Negative Thoughts (ANTs) pop into your head reflexively and seem plausible, even if inaccurate.

- **Recognizing ANTs is the first step:** Identifying your specific ANTs allows you to create distance and realize that thoughts are not facts.

- **The Thought Record is a key tool:** Using a Thought Record helps you capture and analyze your ANTs, emotions, and the cognitive distortions involved.

Chapter 7: Cognitive Restructuring

Challenging and Changing Your Sleep Thoughts

You've spent time identifying your Automatic Negative Thoughts (ANTs) and the cognitive distortions behind them. You're starting to see how your beliefs about sleep fuel the anxiety that keeps you awake. That awareness is a huge step.

But awareness alone is often not enough. If you've held certain beliefs for a long time, they won't disappear just because you recognize they are unhelpful. You need to actively challenge and change them.

This process is called *Cognitive Restructuring*. It's a core technique in Cognitive Behavioral Therapy (CBT). Cognitive restructuring is not just about "positive thinking." It's not about pretending everything is fine when it's not. It's about developing a more realistic, balanced, and helpful perspective. It's about looking at the evidence and testing your beliefs in the real world.

This chapter will equip you with the tools to restructure your sleep-related thoughts. We will explore techniques for challenging your ANTs, developing alternative thoughts, and managing worry. We will also discuss how to let go of the effort to sleep.

Techniques for examining the evidence for and against your sleep-related beliefs

The core of cognitive restructuring is to treat your thoughts as hypotheses—ideas that need to be tested—rather than absolute facts. When you have an automatic negative thought, especially a "hot thought" that causes strong emotion, you need to pause and examine it critically.

Here are some techniques to help you challenge your ANTs and examine the evidence:

1. The Socratic Method (Questioning the Thought)

The Socratic method involves asking a series of questions to explore the validity and usefulness of the thought. Think of yourself as a detective investigating the thought.

Here are some key questions to ask:

- **What is the evidence for this thought?** What facts support it?

- **What is the evidence against this thought?** What facts contradict it? (This is often the most important question, as we tend to ignore evidence that doesn't fit our beliefs).

- **What cognitive distortion is at play here?** (Catastrophizing, All-or-Nothing thinking, etc.)

- **What is the worst that could happen?** And how likely is it?

- **What is the best that could happen?**

- **What is the most likely outcome?**

- **How else could I interpret this situation?** Are there alternative explanations?

- **If a friend had this thought, what would I tell them?** (We are often more compassionate and objective toward others than ourselves).

- **Is this thought helpful?** Does it help me achieve my goals?

Case Example: Challenging a Catastrophic Thought

ANT: "If I don't sleep well tonight, I will bomb my presentation tomorrow." (Catastrophizing)

Questioning the thought:

- **Evidence for:** "I feel tired when I don't sleep well. I might have trouble concentrating."

- **Evidence against:** "I have given presentations on little sleep before and done fine. Adrenaline often kicks in and helps me focus. I know the material well. Even if I'm not at my best, it doesn't mean I will 'bomb' it."

- **Cognitive distortion:** Catastrophizing, All-or-Nothing thinking.

- **Most likely outcome:** "I might feel tired, but I will likely be able to deliver the presentation adequately. It might not be my best performance, but it will be acceptable."

- **Helpful?** "No, this thought is making me anxious, which makes it harder to sleep."

2. Behavioral Experiments

Sometimes the best way to test a belief is to conduct a behavioral experiment. This involves planning a specific activity to test the validity of the belief in the real world.

Example 1: Testing the belief about daytime functioning.

Belief: "If I get less than 6 hours of sleep, I cannot function the next day."

Experiment: After a night of less than 6 hours of sleep, intentionally engage in a demanding cognitive task (e.g., solving a puzzle, writing a report). Rate your performance objectively. Compare it to your prediction.

Result: You might find that while you feel tired, your cognitive performance is not as impaired as you thought. You can still function reasonably well.

Example 2: Testing the belief about others' perception.

Belief: "Everyone can tell when I haven't slept well. I look terrible."

Experiment: After a bad night's sleep, ask a trusted friend or family member how you look.

Result: They might say you look a bit tired, but often they don't notice anything unusual. We tend to overestimate how visible our internal state is to others.

3. Using Sleep Diary Data

Your Sleep Diary provides objective data that can be used to challenge unhelpful beliefs.

Belief: "I never sleep more than 3 hours a night."

Evidence from Sleep Diary: Look at your actual Total Sleep Time (TST) over the past week. You might find that while your sleep is poor, you are actually sleeping more than you perceive (e.g., 5 hours on average).

Belief: "My sleep is getting worse and worse."

Evidence from Sleep Diary: Look at the trend of your Sleep Efficiency (SE) and TST over the weeks you have been implementing CBT-I. You might see gradual improvements that you hadn't noticed.

By consistently examining the evidence, you start to weaken the grip of the automatic negative thoughts. You develop a more realistic and evidence-based perspective.

Developing balanced and helpful thoughts about sleep

Cognitive restructuring is a two-step process. First, you challenge the negative thought. Second, you replace it with a more balanced and helpful alternative thought.

The goal is not to develop overly positive or unrealistic thoughts (e.g., "I will sleep perfectly tonight!"). The goal is to develop thoughts that are accurate, constructive, and reduce anxiety.

Characteristics of Balanced Thoughts:

- **Realistic:** Based on evidence and facts.
- **Helpful:** Promote calmness and reduce arousal.

- **Compassionate:** Kind and understanding toward yourself.

- **Action-oriented (when appropriate):** Focus on what you can control (your behaviors) rather than what you can't (sleep itself).

How to develop alternative thoughts:

Once you have challenged the ANT using the techniques discussed above, summarize the evidence and insights into a balanced thought.

Let's look at some examples of how to replace common cognitive distortions with balanced thoughts:

Distortion: Catastrophizing

- **ANT:** "If I don't sleep well tonight, tomorrow will be ruined."

- **Balanced Thought:** "I might feel tired tomorrow if I don't sleep well, but I can still get through the day. I've handled difficult days before. My day won't be completely ruined."

Distortion: Unrealistic Expectations

- **ANT:** "I must get 8 hours of sleep to function."

- **Balanced Thought:** "While 8 hours might be ideal, I can function reasonably well on less sleep. My sleep needs vary. The goal is improvement, not perfection."

Distortion: Misattribution

- **ANT:** "I'm feeling irritable because of my insomnia."

- **Balanced Thought:** "Lack of sleep might be contributing to my irritability, but stress at work is also a factor. I can take steps to manage my stress, even if I'm tired."

Distortion: All-or-Nothing Thinking

- **ANT:** "If I wake up during the night, the whole night is ruined."

- **Balanced Thought:** "Waking up during the night is normal. I can rest even if I'm awake. I might still get some more sleep before the morning."

Distortion: Fortune Telling

- **ANT:** "I just know I'm going to have a bad night tonight."
- **Balanced Thought:** "I don't know how I will sleep tonight. Sleep is unpredictable. I will focus on my wind-down routine and trust my body's ability to sleep."

The Importance of Practice:

Developing balanced thoughts takes practice. At first, you might find it difficult to come up with alternative thoughts, or you might not fully believe them. That's okay.

The key is to practice consistently. Use the Thought Record to work through the process of challenging and replacing your ANTs. Over time, the balanced thoughts will become more automatic and believable.

Coping Cards:

A useful technique is to write down your most common ANTs and the corresponding balanced thoughts on index cards (Coping Cards). Keep these cards handy (e.g., on your bedside table, in your wallet). When you find yourself struggling with anxiety about sleep, read the coping cards to remind yourself of the balanced perspective.

The technique of "Constructive Worry" (scheduling worry time during the day)

For many people with insomnia, the nighttime is not just filled with worry about sleep. It's also when all the other worries of the day come rushing in. As soon as the distractions of the day fade away, your mind starts racing with concerns about work, family, finances, health, etc.

This nighttime worry creates cognitive arousal that interferes with sleep.

If you try to stop worrying, it usually doesn't work. Telling yourself "Don't worry" is like telling yourself "Don't think of a white bear." It often makes the worry worse.

A more effective strategy is *Constructive Worry*, also known as *Scheduled Worry Time*. This technique, developed by Dr. Thomas Borkovec, helps you manage worry by containing it to a specific time during the day, rather than letting it intrude at night (Borkovec et al., 1983).

How to implement Constructive Worry:

Step 1: Schedule a "Worry Time"

Set aside a specific time each day (e.g., 15-30 minutes) dedicated exclusively to worrying.

- **Timing:** Choose a time that is convenient, but not too close to bedtime (at least 2-3 hours before). Late afternoon or early evening often works well.

- **Location:** Choose a specific place for your worry time (e.g., a desk, a particular chair). Do not do it in bed.

Step 2: Postpone Worry during the Day (and Night)

Throughout the day, when a worry pops into your mind, acknowledge it, but postpone it to your scheduled worry time.

- **Acknowledge:** "That's a worry. I'll think about it during my worry time."

- **Jot it down:** It can be helpful to keep a "Worry List." Write down the worry briefly so you don't forget it.

- **Redirect:** Gently redirect your attention back to the present moment or the task at hand.

The same applies at night. If you find yourself worrying in bed, tell yourself: "This is not the time for worrying. I will think about this tomorrow during my worry time." Then redirect your attention to a relaxation technique or get out of bed if you are awake for too long (Stimulus Control).

Step 3: Engage in Constructive Worry during the Scheduled Time

During your scheduled worry time, sit down and focus on your worries. Don't avoid them.

- **Review your Worry List.**

- **Think about the worries:** Allow yourself to worry.

- **Focus on problem-solving:** This is the "constructive" part. For each worry, ask yourself:

    o "Is this a solvable problem or a hypothetical worry?"

    o If it's solvable, what steps can I take to address it? Brainstorm solutions and develop an action plan.

    o If it's a hypothetical worry (e.g., "What if I get sick?"), acknowledge the uncertainty and practice tolerating it.

Step 4: End the Worry Time

When the time is up, stop worrying. Move on to another activity.

Why Constructive Worry Works:

- **It contains the worry:** By limiting worry to a specific time, you prevent it from spilling over into the rest of your day and night.

- **It reduces cognitive arousal at bedtime:** When you know you have a designated time to address your concerns, you feel less pressure to do it at night.

- **It improves problem-solving:** By focusing on solutions during the day, you address the underlying issues that fuel the worry.

- **It increases your sense of control:** You learn that you can control when and where you worry.

Constructive Worry takes practice. At first, you might find it difficult to postpone worry. But with consistent effort, it becomes easier. It is a powerful tool for reducing nighttime cognitive arousal and improving sleep.

Letting go of the effort to sleep (Paradoxical Intention)

As we discussed earlier, one of the main factors that perpetuates insomnia is *sleep effort*. Trying to force sleep creates tension and arousal that interfere with sleep. Sleep is an involuntary process. You cannot make yourself sleep.

The key to overcoming sleep effort is to let go of the struggle. This is easier said than done, of course. When you are desperate for sleep, it's natural to try hard to achieve it.

Paradoxical Intention is a cognitive technique that helps you let go of sleep effort by doing the opposite of what you are trying to achieve. Instead of trying to fall asleep, you try to stay awake.

It sounds paradoxical (hence the name), but it is an effective strategy for reducing sleep performance anxiety (Espie, 2006).

The Rationale behind Paradoxical Intention:

When you try to stay awake, you remove the pressure to sleep. You stop monitoring your sleepiness and stop worrying about the consequences of not sleeping. This reduces anxiety and arousal, allowing sleep to occur naturally.

Think of it like this: If I tell you, "Don't laugh," you are more likely to laugh. If I tell you, "Try to stay awake," you are more likely to feel sleepy.

How to practice Paradoxical Intention:

1. **Get into bed when sleepy.**

2. **Keep your eyes open (gently):** Lie comfortably in bed with the lights off. Keep your eyes open, focusing gently on a spot in the room.

3. **Tell yourself to stay awake:** Silently repeat phrases like:

   o "I'm going to try to stay awake for as long as possible."

   o "I don't care if I sleep or not."

   o "I'm just going to rest here and stay awake."

4. **Do not engage in stimulating activities:** This is not about actively trying to stay awake by reading or watching TV. It's about passive wakefulness—resting quietly in bed without the intention to sleep.

5. **Allow sleep to happen:** When your eyelids become heavy and you feel yourself drifting off, allow it to happen. Don't resist it.

Important Considerations:

- **It requires practice:** Paradoxical Intention can feel strange at first. It requires a shift in mindset. Practice it consistently.

- **It's not a magic bullet:** It works best when combined with other CBT-I strategies (Stimulus Control, Sleep Restriction, Cognitive Restructuring).

- **Focus on acceptance:** The core of Paradoxical Intention is acceptance. Accepting wakefulness rather than fighting it.

The concept of "Quiet Wakefulness":

Even if you don't practice Paradoxical Intention formally, adopting the mindset of *quiet wakefulness* can be very helpful.

This means recognizing that resting quietly in bed, even if you are awake, is beneficial. It is not a waste of time. It allows your body and mind to rest.

When you find yourself awake at night, instead of feeling frustrated, tell yourself: "It's okay that I'm awake. I'm resting peacefully. Sleep will come when it's ready."

By reducing the pressure to sleep and accepting wakefulness, you create the conditions that allow sleep to emerge naturally.

Workbook Activity: Cognitive Restructuring Exercise (Decatastrophizing and Reappraisal)

Now it's time to put the cognitive restructuring techniques into practice. We will expand the Thought Record you started in the previous chapter by adding new columns to incorporate the challenge and restructuring steps.

(In a physical workbook, a blank expanded Thought Record template would be provided here.)

The Expanded Thought Record:

The expanded Thought Record guides you through the entire process of identifying, challenging, and changing your ANTs. It typically includes 5 or 6 columns.

Columns 1-3: Same as before (Situation/Trigger, ANTs, Emotions and Intensity).

Column 4: Challenge/Evidence

This is where you use the techniques discussed (examining the evidence, questioning the thought, identifying distortions) to critically examine the ANT.

- What is the evidence against this thought?

- What cognitive distortions am I using?

- What would I tell a friend?

Column 5: Balanced/Alternative Thought

This is where you develop a balanced and helpful thought to replace the ANT.

- How can I look at this situation more realistically?

- What is a more helpful thought?

Column 6: Re-rate Emotion Intensity (0-100%)

After developing the balanced thought, re-rate the intensity of the original emotion(s).

- How do I feel now?

Example of a Completed Expanded Thought Record Entry:

Situation: Woke up at 3 AM.

Hot Thought: "Tomorrow will be ruined if I don't get back to sleep."

Emotions: Anxiety (85%), Frustration (90%).

Thinking Distortions: Catastrophizing, fortune-telling.

Challenge/Evidence: In the past, lack of sleep has been uncomfortable but not completely destructive. I was still able to function, and worrying only made it worse.

Balanced Thought: "I can't predict how the night will go. Even if I don't sleep more, I've handled tired days before. I can rest now and use strategies tomorrow—prioritize tasks, take breaks, and manage my energy."

The Goal:

The goal is to reduce the intensity of the negative emotion by changing the underlying thought. Even a small reduction in intensity is progress.

Instructions for the next weeks:

Continue using the Expanded Thought Record daily. Practice challenging and replacing your ANTs.

Decatastrophizing Exercise:

In addition to the Thought Record, practice decatastrophizing your biggest fears about sleep loss.

1. **Identify your biggest fear:** What is the worst consequence of insomnia that you fear? (e.g., "I will lose my job," "I will develop a serious illness").

2. **Assess the likelihood:** How likely is this outcome? (Be realistic, based on evidence).

3. **Develop a coping plan:** If the worst-case scenario did happen, how would you cope with it? What steps would you take?

4. **Reappraise the situation:** Develop a more balanced perspective on the fear.

By confronting your fears directly and developing a plan to cope with them, you reduce their power over you.

Cognitive restructuring is a skill that takes time and effort to master. Be patient and persistent. By changing your thoughts about sleep, you are changing your relationship with sleep, paving the way for lasting improvement.

Changing Sleep Thoughts Summary

- **Cognitive Restructuring challenges unhelpful thoughts:** It involves examining thoughts objectively and developing more realistic perspectives.

- **Examine the evidence:** Treat thoughts as hypotheses. Look for evidence for and against the thought. Ask challenging questions.

- **Conduct behavioral experiments:** Test your beliefs in the real world to gather objective evidence.

- **Develop balanced and helpful thoughts:** Create alternative thoughts that are believable, realistic, and reduce anxiety.

- **Constructive Worry manages daytime worry:** Schedule a specific time during the day to address worries and engage in problem-solving. Postpone worries at night.

- **Paradoxical Intention reduces sleep effort:** Let go of the effort to sleep by trying to stay awake. This reduces performance anxiety and arousal.

- **Embrace quiet wakefulness:** Accept wakefulness and focus on resting rather than struggling.

- **Practice is essential:** Cognitive Restructuring is a skill that requires consistent practice to change ingrained thought patterns.

Chapter 8: Sleep Hygiene - Setting the Stage for Sleep

If you've ever searched online for ways to improve your sleep, you've almost certainly come across the term "sleep hygiene." It's usually the first piece of advice given. Things like keeping your room dark, avoiding caffeine late in the day, and having a comfortable mattress.

These practices are important, for sure. They help create an environment and lifestyle that support healthy sleep. Think of sleep hygiene as setting the stage. If you want a play to be successful, you need good lighting, comfortable seating, and the right props. Sleep hygiene provides the optimal conditions for sleep to occur.

However, here's where things get tricky. If you have chronic insomnia, you've likely already tried many of these things. You bought the blackout curtains, you switched to decaf, you banned your phone from the bedroom. And yet, the insomnia persists. This can be incredibly frustrating. You might think, "My sleep hygiene is perfect, so why can't I sleep?"

This chapter will put sleep hygiene into perspective within the framework of CBT-I. We will look at how your environment and daily habits affect your sleep, and how to optimize them to support the behavioral and cognitive strategies you've been working on.

The role of sleep hygiene in supporting CBT-I (important, but not sufficient alone)

Here is the crucial point about sleep hygiene: **It is necessary, but not sufficient, for treating chronic insomnia.**

Research studies have shown that while sleep hygiene education is helpful for preventing sleep problems and treating mild or short-term sleep difficulties, it is generally ineffective as a standalone treatment for chronic insomnia (Stepanski & Wyatt, 2003).

Why? Because chronic insomnia is primarily driven by stronger factors, such as conditioned arousal (associating the bed with wakefulness), a weakened sleep drive, and cognitive arousal (worry about sleep). Sleep hygiene alone cannot overcome these factors.

If you have trained your brain to be awake in bed, having a perfectly dark room won't fix that association. If you are spending too much time in bed, avoiding caffeine won't be enough to consolidate your sleep.

The Supportive Role of Sleep Hygiene in CBT-I:

In CBT-I, sleep hygiene is used to support the core behavioral and cognitive strategies. It helps remove external factors that might be interfering with sleep, allowing the main strategies to work more effectively.

Think of the core CBT-I strategies (Stimulus Control, Sleep Restriction, Cognitive Restructuring) as the engine that drives sleep improvement. Sleep hygiene is like the oil that keeps the engine running smoothly. You need the engine to move forward, but the oil reduces friction and improves performance.

Important Caveat: Avoid Obsessing over Sleep Hygiene

Be careful not to turn sleep hygiene into another source of anxiety. If you become obsessed with having the perfect conditions for sleep, you can increase arousal and create sleep performance anxiety.

If your room is slightly too warm one night, or if you hear a noise outside, don't panic. Good sleepers can sleep through minor disruptions. The goal is to create a reasonably optimal environment, not a perfect, hermetically sealed sanctuary.

Optimizing your sleep environment (light, noise, temperature)

Your bedroom environment plays a significant role in the quality of your sleep. Your brain relies on environmental cues to regulate the sleep-wake cycle. The ideal sleep environment is **dark, quiet, cool, and comfortable.**

1. Light: The Power of Darkness

Light is the most powerful external cue for regulating your circadian rhythm. Exposure to light at night can disrupt your internal clock and suppress the release of melatonin, the hormone that promotes sleep.

How to optimize light:

- **Blackout curtains or shades:** Use these to block out external light from streetlights and the early morning sun.

- **Eye mask:** If you cannot make your room dark enough, consider using a comfortable eye mask.

- **Dim the lights in the evening:** In the hour or two before bed, dim the lights in your home. Use lamps instead of bright overhead lights.

- **Minimize electronic light:** Avoid using electronic devices (phones, tablets, computers) for at least 1 hour before bedtime. The blue light emitted by these screens is particularly disruptive to melatonin production (Chang et al., 2015).

- **Cover clocks and other LEDs:** Cover or remove any electronic devices in the bedroom that emit light. Remember the rule about not clock-watching!

2. Noise: The Need for Quiet

Noise is a common cause of sleep disruption. Sudden noises can wake you up, and continuous noise can reduce sleep quality.

How to optimize noise:

- **Minimize external noise:** If you live in a noisy area, consider using heavy curtains to muffle the sound.

- **White noise machine or fan:** A consistent, low-level background noise (like a white noise machine or a fan) can help mask disruptive sounds and create a calming environment.

- **Earplugs:** If noise is unavoidable (e.g., a snoring partner, traffic), consider using comfortable earplugs.

- **Address pet disruptions:** If your pets are disrupting your sleep, consider having them sleep in a different room.

3. Temperature: Keeping it Cool

Your body temperature naturally drops in the evening to prepare for sleep. A cool bedroom environment supports this natural process.

How to optimize temperature:

- **Ideal temperature:** Most sleep experts recommend a bedroom temperature between 60-67°F (15-19°C). Experiment to find what is most comfortable for you.

- **Bedding and sleepwear:** Use breathable bedding materials (like cotton or linen). Adjust the layers of your bedding so you can easily regulate your temperature during the night.

- **Warm bath or shower before bed:** Taking a warm bath or shower 1-2 hours before bedtime can help promote sleep. The warmth raises your body temperature, and the subsequent rapid cooldown after getting out signals to your body that it's time to sleep (Haghayegh et al., 2019).

4. Comfort: The Bed Matters

- **Mattress and Pillows:** Ensure your mattress and pillows provide adequate support and comfort. Mattresses generally need to be replaced every 7-10 years.

- **Minimize clutter:** Keep your bedroom clean and uncluttered. A tidy room can promote a sense of calm.

The impact of substances (caffeine, alcohol, nicotine)

What you consume during the day can have a significant impact on your sleep at night.

1. Caffeine: The Alertness Booster (and Sleep Disruptor)

Caffeine is a stimulant that promotes alertness by blocking the action of adenosine (the chemical that builds up sleep pressure).

Impact on sleep:

Caffeine consumption, especially late in the day, can make it harder to fall asleep and decrease the quality of your sleep (Drake et al., 2013).

Key considerations:

- **Half-life:** Caffeine has a relatively long half-life (the time it takes for the body to eliminate half of the substance), typically ranging from 3 to 7 hours. This means that the caffeine from your afternoon coffee might still be circulating in your system at bedtime.

- **Hidden sources:** Be aware of caffeine in soda, tea (including green tea), chocolate, energy drinks, and some medications.

Recommendations:

- **Time it right:** Avoid caffeine in the afternoon and evening. A general guideline is to stop consuming caffeine at least 6-8 hours before bedtime (e.g., before 2 PM). If you are sensitive, you might need an earlier cutoff.

2. Alcohol: The False Friend of Sleep

Alcohol is a central nervous system depressant. It can have a sedative effect, helping you fall asleep faster. However, alcohol significantly disrupts the quality of your sleep later in the night.

Impact on sleep:

- **Fragmented sleep:** As the alcohol is metabolized, it causes a "rebound effect," leading to frequent awakenings and shallow sleep in the second half of the night.

- **Suppression of REM sleep:** Alcohol suppresses REM sleep (the dreaming stage).

- **Worsening of sleep apnea:** Alcohol relaxes the muscles in the throat, which can worsen snoring and sleep apnea.

Recommendations:

- **Avoid alcohol as a sleep aid:** Do not rely on alcohol to help you sleep. It ultimately makes the problem worse.

- **Time it right:** If you choose to drink, avoid alcohol within 3-4 hours of bedtime to allow time for it to be metabolized.

3. Nicotine: The Hidden Stimulant

Nicotine (found in cigarettes and vaping products) is also a stimulant. It increases heart rate, blood pressure, and brain activity.

Impact on sleep:

Nicotine use close to bedtime can make it harder to fall asleep. Furthermore, nicotine withdrawal symptoms (like cravings) can occur during the night, leading to awakenings.

Recommendations:

- **Quit smoking/vaping:** This is the best strategy for improving your sleep and overall health.

- **Avoid nicotine before bed:** If you use nicotine products, avoid using them close to bedtime or during the night.

The role of exercise and diet

Your overall lifestyle habits also play a role in regulating your sleep.

1. Exercise: The Natural Sleep Promoter

Regular physical activity is one of the best things you can do for your sleep. Exercise promotes healthy sleep by increasing sleep drive, reducing stress, and improving sleep quality (Kredlow et al., 2015).

Recommendations:

- **Be consistent:** Aim for at least 30 minutes of moderate-intensity exercise most days of the week.

- **Timing:** The best time to exercise is in the morning or early afternoon.

What about exercising in the evening?

Recent research suggests that moderate-intensity exercise in the evening does not negatively affect sleep for most people, as long as it is completed at least 1-2 hours before bedtime (Stutz et al., 2019). However, vigorous exercise close to bedtime might still be disruptive for some individuals. Pay attention to how your body responds.

2. Diet: Eating for Sleep

While there is no magic diet for sleep, your eating habits can affect your sleep quality.

Recommendations:

- **Avoid large meals close to bedtime:** Eating a heavy meal close to bedtime can cause discomfort and indigestion. Allow at least 2-3 hours between your last meal and bedtime.

- **Limit fluid intake in the evening:** Reduce your fluid intake in the evening to minimize awakenings to use the bathroom (*nocturia*).

- **Light snack if needed:** If you feel hungry before bed, a light snack (e.g., whole-grain crackers with cheese, or a banana) might be helpful. Avoid sugary snacks.

Developing a relaxing pre-sleep routine

A consistent pre-sleep routine is essential for winding down and signaling to your brain that it's time to transition from wakefulness to sleep. It acts as a buffer zone between the stress of the day and the calm of the night.

How to develop a pre-sleep routine:

1. **Set a consistent time:** Start your routine at the same time every evening, about 30-60 minutes before your intended bedtime.

2. **Transition away from stimulating activities:**
   - Turn off the TV and computer.
   - Put away your work or studies.
   - Avoid emotional or stressful conversations.

3. **Engage in relaxing activities:** Choose activities that you find calming and enjoyable.
   - Reading a book (on the couch or a chair, not in bed).
   - Listening to calming music, an audiobook, or a podcast.
   - Practicing relaxation techniques (covered in the next chapter).
   - Gentle stretching or yoga.
   - Taking a warm bath or shower.

4. **Keep the lights dim:** Perform your routine in a dimly lit environment.

Workbook Activity: Sleep Hygiene Checklist and Action Plan

Now it's time to evaluate your current sleep hygiene practices and develop a plan for improvement.

(In a physical workbook, this section would include a checklist and a worksheet for planning.)

Part 1: Sleep Hygiene Checklist

Review the following checklist and identify areas where you can make improvements.

Environment:

[ ] My bedroom is dark.

[ ] My bedroom is quiet.

[ ] My bedroom is cool (60-67°F / 15-19°C).

[ ] My bed is comfortable.

Substances:

[ ] I avoid caffeine in the afternoon and evening.

[ ] I avoid alcohol within 3-4 hours of bedtime.

[ ] I avoid nicotine before bedtime.

Lifestyle:

[ ] I exercise regularly.

[ ] I avoid large meals close to bedtime.

[ ] I limit fluid intake in the evening.

Routine:

[ ] I have a consistent relaxing pre-sleep routine (30-60 minutes).

[ ] I avoid electronic devices for at least 1 hour before bed.

[ ] I dim the lights in the evening.

Part 2: Action Plan

Based on your checklist, identify 2-3 specific changes you will make this week. Focus on the changes that are most likely to have an impact.

Be specific and realistic.

Example:

Goal 1 (Caffeine): "I will switch from regular coffee to decaf after 12 PM every day."

Goal 2 (Routine): "I will stop using my phone 30 minutes before bedtime and read a book instead, starting tonight."

Remember, the goal is improvement, not perfection. Implement these changes gradually and consistently.

Sleep Hygiene Fundamentals

- **Necessary but not sufficient:** Good sleep hygiene supports sleep but does not treat the core drivers of chronic insomnia.

- **Optimize the environment:** Create a sleep environment that is dark, quiet, cool, and comfortable.

- **Manage substances:** Be mindful of the impact of caffeine, alcohol, and nicotine. Avoid them in the hours before bedtime.

- **Healthy lifestyle habits:** Engage in regular exercise and maintain healthy eating habits.

- **Develop a relaxing pre-sleep routine:** Create a consistent wind-down routine in the hour before bed to help you transition to sleep.

- **Balance is key:** Implement sleep hygiene practices without becoming overly rigid or anxious about them.

Chapter 9: Relaxation and Mindfulness Techniques

We have covered the behavioral and cognitive strategies of CBT-I. But what about the physical tension and arousal that often accompany insomnia? The tight muscles, the racing heart, the feeling of being "on edge"?

This chapter focuses on the final component of the CBT-I toolkit: Relaxation Techniques. These techniques are designed to directly counteract the physiological and cognitive arousal that interferes with sleep.

Relaxation is not just about feeling calm. It's about actively triggering a physiological response that is the opposite of the stress response.

The relaxation response and its role in reducing arousal

Your autonomic nervous system has two main modes: the "Fight-or-Flight" response (sympathetic nervous system) and the "Rest-and-Digest" response (parasympathetic nervous system).

In chronic insomnia, the fight-or-flight system is often overactive, leading to hyperarousal.

The *Relaxation Response*, a term coined by Dr. Herbert Benson, is the physiological state induced by the activation of the parasympathetic nervous system (Benson et al., 1974). It is a state of deep rest characterized by slower breathing, lower heart rate, reduced muscle tension, and a calmer mental state.

The Role in Insomnia Treatment:

By learning to activate the Relaxation Response, you can directly reduce the arousal that interferes with sleep.

Important Considerations for Using Relaxation Techniques:

1. Relaxation is a skill:

Learning to relax is a skill that requires practice. Don't expect immediate results. It takes time to train your body and mind.

2. Practice during the day:

It is crucial to practice these techniques during the day, when you are relatively calm. This makes it easier to use them effectively at night when you are anxious. Aim for 10-20 minutes of practice daily.

3. The goal is relaxation, not sleep:

This is a very important point. Do not use relaxation techniques as a way to force sleep. If you try to use them to make yourself fall asleep, you are engaging in sleep effort, which can backfire by increasing anxiety. Focus on the process of relaxation, and let sleep come naturally.

4. Find what works for you:

Experiment with the different methods presented in this chapter and find the ones that resonate with you.

Let's explore some specific techniques.

Progressive Muscle Relaxation (PMR) script and practice

Progressive Muscle Relaxation (PMR) involves systematically tensing and then releasing different muscle groups throughout the body.

The Rationale:

PMR helps you become aware of the difference between tension and relaxation. By intentionally tensing the muscles and then releasing the tension, you can induce a state of deep physical relaxation, which in turn calms the mind.

How to practice PMR:

PMR involves a sequence of tensing and releasing muscle groups.

1. **Preparation:** Find a comfortable position. Close your eyes. Take a few deep breaths.

2. **Tensing:** Focus on a specific muscle group. Tense the muscles firmly but gently. Hold the tension for about 5 seconds.

3. **Releasing:** Quickly release the tension. Focus on the feeling of relaxation. Pause for about 10-15 seconds.

4. **Progression:** Move systematically through the different muscle groups.

PMR Script (Short Version):

Here is a short PMR script that you can follow.

(Start with a few deep breaths.)

1. Hands and Forearms:

Tense: Clench your hands into fists. Hold (5 seconds).

Release: Relax your hands completely. Feel the tension melting away. (10-15 seconds).

2. Biceps and Upper Arms:

Tense: Bend your elbows and flex your biceps. Hold (5 seconds).

Release: Straighten your arms and let them rest comfortably. (10-15 seconds).

3. Shoulders:

Tense: Shrug your shoulders up toward your ears. Hold (5 seconds).

Release: Let your shoulders drop down completely. (10-15 seconds).

4. Face (Forehead, Eyes, Jaw):

Tense: Wrinkle your forehead, squeeze your eyes shut tightly, and clench your jaw. Hold (5 seconds).

Release: Relax your forehead, let your eyelids rest gently, and unclench your jaw. (10-15 seconds).

5. Chest and Stomach:

Tense: Take a deep breath and hold it, tensing your chest and stomach muscles. Hold (5 seconds).

Release: Exhale slowly and let your chest and stomach relax completely. (10-15 seconds).

6. Hips and Buttocks:

Tense: Squeeze your buttocks muscles together. Hold (5 seconds).

Release: Relax the muscles completely. (10-15 seconds).

7. Thighs and Legs:

Tense: Straighten your legs and point your toes toward your head, tensing your thigh muscles. Hold (5 seconds).

Release: Relax your legs completely. Feel the heaviness and relaxation. (10-15 seconds).

8. Final Relaxation:

Scan your entire body for any remaining tension. Enjoy the feeling of deep relaxation for a few minutes.

Diaphragmatic (Belly) Breathing exercises

Diaphragmatic Breathing, also known as belly breathing or deep breathing, is a simple yet powerful technique for activating the Relaxation Response.

The Rationale:

When stressed, breathing tends to become shallow and rapid (chest breathing). Diaphragmatic breathing involves taking slow, deep breaths that engage the diaphragm. This type of breathing stimulates the vagus nerve, which plays a key role in calming the nervous system (Gerritsen & Band, 2018).

How to practice Diaphragmatic Breathing:

1. **Preparation:** Sit or lie down comfortably.

2. **Positioning:** Place one hand on your chest and the other hand on your belly.

3. **Inhale:** Inhale slowly and deeply through your nose. As you inhale, your belly should expand outwards. The hand on your belly should rise, while the hand on your chest should remain relatively still.

4. **Exhale:** Exhale slowly and completely through your mouth (or nose). As you exhale, let your belly relax inwards.

5. **Rhythm:** Continue breathing slowly and smoothly. Aim for a slow rhythm (e.g., inhale for 4 counts, pause for 1 count, exhale for 4-6 counts).

Variations:

- **4-7-8 Breathing:** Inhale for 4 counts, hold the breath for 7 counts, and exhale for 8 counts. Repeat the cycle for 4 breaths. (If holding your breath is uncomfortable, skip this variation).

- **Coherent Breathing:** Inhale for 5 seconds, exhale for 5 seconds. This steady rate helps balance the nervous system.

Deep breathing is a versatile tool. You can practice it anytime, anywhere.

Guided imagery and visualization

Guided Imagery, or visualization, is a technique that uses the power of imagination to create a calm and peaceful mental state.

The Rationale:

When you imagine yourself in a relaxing environment, your body responds as if you were actually there, triggering the Relaxation Response. Guided imagery also helps shift your attention away from racing thoughts and worries.

How to practice Guided Imagery:

1. **Preparation:** Find a comfortable position. Close your eyes. Start with a few deep breaths.

2. **Choose a scene:** Choose a place that you find deeply relaxing (e.g., a beach, a forest, a mountain meadow).

3. **Engage your senses:** Imagine this scene in vivid detail.

    o   **Sight:** What do you see?

    o   **Sound:** What do you hear?

    o   **Smell:** What do you smell?

    o   **Touch:** What do you feel on your skin?

4. **Immerse yourself:** Allow yourself to become fully immersed in the scene. Feel the sense of calm and peace spreading through your body.

Guided Imagery Resources:

While you can practice visualization on your own, many people find it helpful to listen to guided imagery recordings.

Mindfulness meditation for sleep (Body Scan, Mindfulness of Thoughts)

Mindfulness Meditation is a practice that involves focusing your attention on the present moment, non-judgmentally. It involves observing your thoughts, feelings, and bodily sensations without getting caught up in them.

The Rationale:

Mindfulness helps address the cognitive arousal that fuels insomnia. You learn to observe your thoughts without reacting to them. Mindfulness also promotes acceptance of the present moment, including wakefulness, reducing the struggle and frustration associated with insomnia (Black et al., 2015).

Here are two mindfulness practices that are particularly helpful for sleep:

1. Body Scan Meditation

The Body Scan involves systematically bringing attention to different parts of the body, noticing sensations without trying to change them.

How to practice the Body Scan:

1. **Preparation:** Lie down comfortably. Close your eyes.
2. **Scan the body:** Start at your feet. Bring your attention to the sensations in this area (e.g., warmth, tingling, pressure).
3. **Move systematically:** Slowly move your attention up through your body—legs, hips, torso, arms, shoulders, neck, and head.
4. **Acknowledge sensations:** As you focus on each part, acknowledge the sensations present. If you notice tension, gently breathe into it, without forcing it to relax.
5. **If the mind wanders:** When your mind wanders, gently guide your attention back to the body part you were focusing on.

The Body Scan promotes deep physical relaxation and increases body awareness.

2. Mindfulness of Thoughts (Observing the Mind)

This practice involves observing your thoughts as they arise and pass away, without getting entangled in them.

How to practice Mindfulness of Thoughts:

1. **Preparation:** Sit or lie down comfortably.

2. **Focus on the breath:** Start by focusing on your breath as an anchor.

3. **Observe thoughts:** As thoughts arise, acknowledge them without judgment.

4. **Visualize the thoughts:** It can be helpful to use a visualization.

   o **Leaves on a stream:** Imagine your thoughts as leaves floating down a stream. Observe them as they appear, float by, and disappear.

   o **Clouds in the sky:** Imagine your thoughts as clouds passing through the sky.

5. **Return to the breath:** Gently guide your attention back to the breath.

This practice helps you realize that you are not your thoughts. This reduces the power of the thoughts to create anxiety and arousal.

Workbook Activity: Relaxation Practice Log

Implementing relaxation techniques requires consistent practice. This activity will help you plan and track your relaxation practice.

(In a physical workbook, this section would include a practice log template.)

1. Experiment and Choose:

Over the next week, experiment with the different relaxation techniques discussed. Try each technique at least twice.

2. Plan your Practice:

Develop a plan for incorporating relaxation practice into your daily routine.

- **Daytime Practice:** Schedule at least one 10-15 minute practice session during the day.

- **Pre-Sleep Routine:** Incorporate a relaxation technique into your wind-down routine.

- **Nighttime Practice:** Plan which technique you will use if you are having trouble falling asleep or if you wake up during the night.

3. Relaxation Practice Log:

Use a log to track your daily practice and observe the effects.

Example – Completed for One Week

Day	Technique Used	Duration (min)	Time of Day/Night	Relaxation Level Before (0–10)	Relaxation Level After (0–10)	Notes/Observations
Mon	Deep breathing	10	Evening, before bed	3	6	Felt calmer, took less time to fall asleep.
Tue	Progressive muscle relaxation	15	Night, in bed	2	7	Helped reduce tension in shoulders.
Wed	Guided imagery	12	Afternoon break	4	8	Mind drifted, but overall calming.
Thu	Body scan	20	Evening	5	7	Noticed areas of tension I usually ignore.
Fri	Gentle stretching	10	Morning	3	6	Helped ease stiffness; mood improved.
Sat	Meditation (mindfulness)	15	Afternoon	4	8	Attention wandered, but I refocused.
Sun	Soothing music	30	Evening	3	7	Relaxed; drifted into light nap.

Remember the goal: The goal is relaxation, not sleep. Focus on the process and the feeling of calm.

Relaxation and Mindfulness Insights

- **The Relaxation Response counteracts stress:** Activating the Relaxation Response reduces physiological and cognitive arousal.

- **Relaxation is a skill:** It requires regular practice. Practice during the day to develop the skill.

- **The goal is relaxation, not sleep:** Avoid using these techniques to force sleep, as this creates sleep effort.

- **Progressive Muscle Relaxation (PMR):** Systematically tensing and releasing muscle groups to induce physical relaxation.

- **Diaphragmatic Breathing:** Slow, deep belly breathing calms the nervous system.

- **Guided Imagery:** Using imagination to create a calming scene reduces arousal and distracts from worries.

- **Mindfulness Meditation:** Focusing on the present moment non-judgmentally helps reduce cognitive arousal and promotes acceptance.

Chapter 10: Troubleshooting Common Challenges

You've been working hard. You've changed your habits, adjusted your sleep schedule, and tackled those unhelpful thoughts. Hopefully, you are starting to see real improvements in your sleep. But let's be real. The journey to better sleep is rarely a straight line. It's more like a winding road, with ups and downs, unexpected detours, and maybe a few potholes.

This is completely normal. Life happens. Stress returns. You get sick. You travel. You might have a few bad nights and feel like you're backsliding.

This chapter is about navigating those challenges. It's your troubleshooting guide. We will discuss how to handle setbacks, manage external disruptions, address co-occurring conditions, and navigate the process of reducing sleep medications.

The key is to approach these challenges with the same skills and strategies you've learned throughout this workbook: flexibility, persistence, and self-compassion.

Dealing with "bad nights" and setbacks

It's inevitable. Even the best sleepers have bad nights sometimes. When you are recovering from chronic insomnia, a bad night can feel particularly discouraging. You might worry that the insomnia is returning, or that the CBT-I strategies have stopped working.

This fear can trigger the old patterns of anxiety and cognitive arousal. You might start catastrophizing: "Oh no, I'm back to square one." This reaction can turn a single bad night into a prolonged setback.

The Difference Between a Lapse and a Relapse:

It's important to distinguish between a *lapse* and a *relapse*.

- A *lapse* (or setback) is a temporary return to old patterns or a brief period of poor sleep. It might last a few nights or even a week. It is often triggered by a specific event (stress, illness).

- A *relapse* is a full return to chronic insomnia patterns over a longer period.

A lapse does not have to become a relapse. How you respond to the setback makes all the difference.

Strategies for Handling a Bad Night:

Here is a step-by-step guide to managing a bad night without letting it derail your progress:

1. Normalize the Experience:

Remind yourself that occasional bad nights are normal. They do not mean you have failed or that the insomnia is back. Sleep is naturally variable.

2. Practice Acceptance (The Cognitive Shift):

Instead of fighting the wakefulness, practice acceptance. Use the cognitive restructuring techniques you learned.

- *Unhelpful Thought:* "I can't believe this is happening again. I'll never get better."

- *Balanced Thought:* "This is just one bad night. It's frustrating, but I can handle it. I have the tools to manage it."

Focus on quiet wakefulness—resting peacefully without the pressure to sleep.

3. Stick to the Rules (The Behavioral Anchor):

This is the most crucial step. When you have a bad night, it is tempting to abandon the CBT-I strategies in an effort to get more sleep. You might want to sleep in late, take a long nap, or spend extra time in bed.

Do not do this. These behaviors are the perpetuating factors that maintain insomnia. They might provide temporary relief, but they will disrupt your sleep drive and circadian rhythm, making the problem worse in the long run.

- **Maintain your Consistent Wake Time:** Get out of bed at your scheduled time, no matter how little you slept. This is hard, I know. But it is essential for building sleep drive for the next night.

- **Follow Stimulus Control:** If you are awake for more than 15-20 minutes, get out of bed. Do something relaxing and return only when sleepy.

- **Avoid Napping:** Resist the urge to nap during the day.

4. Analyze the Cause (Be a Sleep Detective):

The next day, reflect on what might have contributed to the bad night.

- Was there a specific trigger? (Stress, illness, argument?)

- Did you deviate from your routine? (Caffeine late in the day, alcohol, irregular schedule?)

- Were you experiencing increased cognitive arousal? (Worry, racing thoughts?)

Identifying the cause helps you understand the setback and develop a plan to address it. But don't obsess over finding a cause. Sometimes, bad nights just happen for no apparent reason.

5. Focus on What You Can Control:

You cannot control sleep directly. But you can control your behaviors and your responses. Focus on consistently applying the CBT-I strategies. Trust the process.

Case Example: Maria's Setback

Maria had been doing well with CBT-I for six weeks. Her sleep had improved significantly. Then, she had a stressful week at work and started waking up in the middle of the night again. She felt anxious and discouraged.

Maria's response:

Instead of panicking, Maria recognized this as a setback triggered by stress. She continued to get up at 6 AM every morning, even though she felt exhausted. When she woke up at night, she got out of bed and read in the living room until she felt sleepy. She also dedicated time during the day to practice relaxation techniques and used the Constructive Worry technique to address her work stress. After a few days, her sleep started to improve again. She avoided a full relapse by sticking to the rules and managing her anxiety.

Managing external disruptions (noise, travel, illness)

Life is full of disruptions that can interfere with sleep. While we cannot eliminate them entirely, we can develop strategies to manage their impact.

1. Noise:

We discussed optimizing your sleep environment in Chapter 8. If noise continues to be a problem:

- **Masking:** Use a white noise machine or earplugs consistently.

- **Cognitive Reappraisal:** How you perceive the noise matters. If you view the noise as a threat or an unbearable intrusion, it will create arousal. Try to reappraise the noise as neutral background sound.

2. Travel and Jet Lag:

Travel, especially across time zones, disrupts your circadian rhythm, leading to jet lag.

Strategies for Managing Travel:

- **Adjust gradually:** A few days before your trip, gradually adjust your sleep schedule closer to the destination time zone (if feasible).

- **Hydrate:** Drink plenty of water during the flight. Avoid alcohol and caffeine.

- **Light exposure:** When you arrive, use light exposure to help reset your internal clock.

  ○ *Traveling East:* Get bright light in the morning and avoid light in the evening.

  ○ *Traveling West:* Get bright light in the evening and avoid light in the morning.

- **Maintain consistency (as much as possible):** Try to maintain a consistent wake time and pre-sleep routine in the new location.

- **Strategic use of Melatonin:** Melatonin supplements might help adjust your internal clock faster. Consult with your doctor about the appropriate dosage and timing.

3. Illness:

When you are sick (e.g., cold, flu, pain), your sleep is often disrupted. This is normal. Your body needs rest to recover.

Strategies for Managing Illness:

- **Allow for extra rest (but not excessive time in bed):** It's okay to rest more when you are sick. However, try to avoid spending the entire day in bed.

- **Maintain some routine:** Try to maintain a somewhat regular sleep schedule if possible.

- **Address symptoms:** Use medications to manage symptoms (fever, congestion, pain) that might interfere with sleep.

- **Resume CBT-I strategies as soon as possible:** Once you start feeling better, return to your regular sleep schedule and CBT-I practices immediately. Don't let the illness become a trigger for a prolonged setback.

4. Shift Work:

If you work irregular hours or night shifts, maintaining a consistent sleep schedule is extremely challenging. Shift work forces you to sleep against your natural circadian rhythm.

While CBT-I strategies can still be helpful, shift work requires specialized strategies focusing on light exposure, napping, and managing the circadian misalignment. If you are a shift worker, consider consulting with a sleep specialist for personalized guidance.

Insomnia and co-occurring conditions (brief overview of pain, anxiety, depression)

Insomnia rarely occurs in isolation. It often co-exists with other medical or mental health conditions. These conditions can trigger or worsen insomnia, and insomnia can, in turn, exacerbate the symptoms of these conditions. It's a complex bidirectional relationship.

It is crucial to address these co-occurring conditions effectively to achieve lasting improvement in your sleep.

1. Chronic Pain:

Chronic pain (e.g., arthritis, back pain, fibromyalgia) is a common cause of sleep disruption. Pain makes it difficult to fall asleep and can cause frequent awakenings. Poor sleep, in turn, can increase pain sensitivity (Finan et al., 2013).

Management:

- **Optimize pain management:** Work with your healthcare provider to develop an effective pain management plan, including medication, physical therapy, or other interventions.

- **CBT for Pain (CBT-P):** Cognitive Behavioral Therapy for Pain is an effective treatment that helps change how you perceive and respond to pain.

- **Adapt CBT-I:** CBT-I strategies can be adapted for people with chronic pain. For example, if getting out of bed (Stimulus Control) is difficult due to pain, you can modify the rule to sit up in bed or focus on quiet wakefulness.

2. Anxiety Disorders:

Anxiety and insomnia go hand-in-hand. Anxiety causes hyperarousal, which interferes with sleep. Insomnia can increase anxiety levels.

Management:

- **CBT-I addresses sleep-related anxiety:** The cognitive restructuring techniques in CBT-I directly address the worry and anxiety related to sleep.

- **Treat the underlying anxiety:** If you have a generalized anxiety disorder, panic disorder, or PTSD, it is important to seek treatment for the anxiety itself (e.g., Cognitive Behavioral Therapy, medication).

- **Relaxation techniques:** The relaxation and mindfulness techniques discussed in Chapter 9 are particularly helpful for managing anxiety.

3. Depression:

The relationship between insomnia and depression is strong. Insomnia is a common symptom of depression, and people with insomnia are at higher risk of developing depression (Baglioni et al., 2011).

Management:

- **Treat the depression:** Seek professional help for depression (e.g., psychotherapy, medication).

- **CBT-I can improve depression symptoms:** Research has shown that treating insomnia with CBT-I can also lead to improvements in depression symptoms (Manber et al., 2008).

- **Behavioral activation:** Engaging in enjoyable and meaningful activities during the day (behavioral activation) is a key component of depression treatment and can also improve sleep.

4. Other Sleep Disorders:

Sometimes, insomnia is caused or complicated by other underlying sleep disorders.

- **Sleep Apnea:** This condition involves repeated pauses in breathing during sleep, leading to fragmented sleep and daytime sleepiness. If you snore loudly, gasp for air during sleep, or have excessive daytime sleepiness, talk to your doctor about getting tested for sleep apnea.

- **Restless Legs Syndrome (RLS):** This condition involves an uncomfortable urge to move the legs, especially in the evening, which can interfere with falling asleep.

If you suspect you might have another sleep disorder, it is essential to consult with a sleep specialist for proper diagnosis and treatment.

The Importance of Professional Consultation:

If you have a co-occurring medical or mental health condition, it is important to work with your healthcare providers to develop an integrated treatment plan. While this workbook provides valuable tools for managing insomnia, it is not a substitute for professional medical advice.

The role of sleep medications and strategies for reduction (in consultation with a healthcare provider)

Many people with chronic insomnia use prescription or over-the-counter (OTC) sleep aids. If you are currently taking sleep medication, you might be wondering how it fits into the CBT-I program.

The Role of Sleep Medications:

- **Short-term relief:** Sleep medications can be helpful for short-term insomnia (e.g., during periods of acute stress or travel).

- **Not a long-term solution:** Sleep medications do not address the underlying causes of chronic insomnia. They are a band-aid.

- **Potential downsides:** Long-term use of sleep medications can lead to tolerance (needing higher doses for the same effect), dependence (difficulty sleeping without them), and side effects (e.g., daytime drowsiness, memory problems).

CBT-I and Sleep Medications:

CBT-I is the recommended first-line treatment for chronic insomnia because it is more effective than medication in the long term (Mitchell et al., 2012).

The goal of CBT-I is to equip you with the skills to sleep well without relying on medication. Many people who complete CBT-I are able to reduce or eliminate their use of sleep aids.

Strategies for Reducing Sleep Medications:

If you want to reduce your use of sleep medication, it is crucial to do so gradually and in consultation with your healthcare provider.

Important Disclaimer: Do not stop taking prescription sleep medication suddenly ("cold turkey"). This can cause withdrawal symptoms and rebound insomnia (a temporary worsening of sleep). Always consult with your doctor before making any changes to your medication regimen.

Here are the general principles for reducing sleep medication while engaging in CBT-I:

1. Implement CBT-I strategies first:

Start implementing the behavioral and cognitive strategies of CBT-I before attempting to reduce your medication. This allows you to build up your sleep skills and confidence.

2. Gradual Tapering:

The process of reducing medication is called tapering. It involves gradually decreasing the dosage or frequency of the medication over several weeks or months.

- **Dosage reduction:** If you take medication daily, your doctor might recommend gradually reducing the dose (e.g., cutting the pill in half).

- **Frequency reduction:** Alternatively, your doctor might recommend reducing the number of nights you take the medication (e.g., taking it every other night).

3. Monitor your progress:

Continue tracking your sleep using the Sleep Diary during the tapering process. This helps you and your doctor monitor the impact of the medication reduction.

4. Expect some disruption:

As you reduce the medication, you might experience some temporary increase in sleep difficulties (rebound insomnia). This is normal. Use the CBT-I strategies to manage these disruptions.

5. Be patient and flexible:

The tapering process takes time. Be patient with yourself. If you experience significant difficulty, your doctor might slow down the tapering schedule.

Case Example: James's Medication Reduction

James had been taking a prescription sleep aid every night for five years. He started CBT-I and was motivated to stop relying on the medication.

The process:

After four weeks of implementing Stimulus Control and Sleep Restriction, James's sleep efficiency improved. He consulted with his doctor, who developed a tapering plan.

Weeks 1-2: James reduced his dose by half every night.

Weeks 3-4: He took the half dose every other night.

Weeks 5-6: He took the half dose two nights a week.

Week 7: He stopped the medication completely.

During the tapering process, James experienced a few nights of increased wakefulness. He used the CBT-I strategies (getting out of bed, cognitive restructuring) to cope. By the end of the process, he was sleeping well without medication.

What about Over-the-Counter (OTC) Sleep Aids?

OTC sleep aids (e.g., those containing antihistamines) are generally not recommended for long-term use. They can cause side effects and their effectiveness is limited. The same principles of gradual reduction apply to OTC sleep aids.

By combining CBT-I with a structured medication reduction plan (under medical supervision), you can successfully transition away from reliance on sleep aids and achieve sustainable, healthy sleep.

Troubleshooting Guideposts

- **Setbacks are normal:** Occasional bad nights (lapses) are a normal part of the recovery process. Do not let them turn into a relapse.

- **Stick to the rules:** When you have a bad night, it is crucial to maintain your consistent wake time, follow Stimulus Control, and avoid napping.

- **Manage disruptions proactively:** Develop strategies to manage external disruptions like noise, travel, and illness.

- **Address co-occurring conditions:** Insomnia often co-exists with conditions like pain, anxiety, and depression. Treating these conditions is essential for improving sleep.

- **Consult professionals:** If you suspect another sleep disorder or have a co-occurring condition, seek professional help.

- **Medication reduction requires a plan:** If you want to reduce sleep medication, do so gradually and in consultation with your healthcare provider. Implement CBT-I strategies first.

Chapter 11: Relapse Prevention and Long-Term Sleep Health

Congratulations. You have reached the final chapter of this workbook. You have put in a tremendous amount of effort over the past several weeks. You have changed long-standing habits, challenged unhelpful beliefs, and developed new skills for managing your sleep.

You should feel proud of your progress.

But the journey doesn't end here. CBT-I is not just a short-term fix. It's about creating lasting change and maintaining healthy sleep for life.

This final chapter focuses on *Relapse Prevention*. We will review your progress, identify potential risks for future sleep problems, and develop a personalized plan for maintaining your gains and handling any recurrence of insomnia symptoms.

The goal is to empower you to become your own sleep coach.

Reviewing your progress and celebrating successes

The first step in maintaining your progress is to acknowledge how far you have come. When you are focused on the day-to-day challenges, it's easy to lose sight of the overall improvement.

1. Review your Sleep Diaries:

Look back at your baseline Sleep Diary from the beginning of the program. Compare it to your most recent Sleep Diary.

- How has your Sleep Efficiency (SE) changed?

- How has your Total Sleep Time (TST) changed?

- How has the time it takes you to fall asleep (Sleep Latency) changed?

- How has the time you spend awake during the night (WASO) changed?

Seeing the objective data can be very motivating and reinforcing.

2. Re-take the Insomnia Severity Index (ISI):

Complete the ISI questionnaire again (from Chapter 3). Compare your current score to your baseline score.

3. Reflect on Daytime Functioning:

Beyond the numbers, reflect on how your daily life has changed.

- How is your energy level?

- How is your mood?

- How is your concentration and productivity?

- Are you engaging in activities you enjoy?

4. Acknowledge the Behavioral and Cognitive Changes:

Reflect on the changes you have made in your habits and thinking patterns.

- Are you maintaining a consistent sleep schedule?

- Are you using the bed only for sleep?

- Are you challenging unhelpful thoughts about sleep?

- Are you practicing relaxation techniques?

Celebrate Your Successes:

Take time to celebrate your achievements. You have tackled a challenging problem and made significant improvements in your health and well-being.

Acknowledge the effort and persistence it took to get here. Celebrating your success reinforces your commitment to maintaining these changes.

Identifying high-risk situations for relapse

While CBT-I provides lasting skills, it does not make you immune to future sleep problems. Life will continue to present challenges that can disrupt your sleep.

The key to relapse prevention is to identify the situations that put you at high risk for a recurrence of insomnia symptoms. These are your personal triggers.

Common High-Risk Situations:

- **Stress:** This is the most common trigger for insomnia relapse. Major life changes (e.g., job change, moving, relationship difficulties), increased workload, financial stress, or grief can all disrupt sleep.

- **Illness or Injury:** Medical problems, especially those causing pain or discomfort, can interfere with sleep.

- **Travel:** Traveling across time zones disrupts the circadian rhythm.

- **Changes in Routine:** Changes in your work schedule, having a new baby, or other disruptions to your daily routine can affect your sleep.

- **Periods of Low Mood or Anxiety:** Mental health challenges can trigger a return of insomnia symptoms.

Identifying Your Personal Triggers:

Reflect on your past experiences with insomnia.

- What triggered your insomnia initially (the Precipitating factors)?

- What situations have caused setbacks during the program?

- What areas of your life are most likely to cause stress in the future?

By identifying your high-risk situations, you can prepare for them proactively.

Recognizing Early Warning Signs:

Relapse rarely happens overnight. There are usually early warning signs that indicate your sleep is starting to deteriorate.

Common Early Warning Signs:

- Difficulty falling asleep for a few consecutive nights.

- Increased awakenings during the night.

- Waking up earlier than usual.

- Increased worry or anxiety about sleep.

- Feeling more tired or irritable during the day.

- Slipping back into old habits (e.g., spending more time in bed, irregular schedule, increased caffeine use).

Recognizing these early warning signs allows you to intervene early before a full relapse occurs.

Developing a long-term sleep maintenance plan

Maintaining healthy sleep requires ongoing effort. It's like maintaining physical fitness. You cannot exercise for a few weeks and expect to stay fit for the rest of your life. You need to incorporate healthy habits into your lifestyle.

Your long-term sleep maintenance plan should include the following components:

1. Maintaining Healthy Sleep Behaviors:

The behavioral strategies you learned are the foundation of healthy sleep. Continue practicing them consistently.

- **Consistent Sleep Schedule:** Maintain a regular wake time, 7 days a week. Allow for some flexibility (e.g., sleeping in 30-60 minutes on weekends), but avoid large variations.

- **Optimal Sleep Window:** Find the sleep window that allows you to achieve high Sleep Efficiency (85% or higher) and feel refreshed during the day. Adjust it if needed.

- **Stimulus Control:** Continue using the bed only for sleep and sex. If you find yourself awake in bed, get up.

- **Healthy Lifestyle:** Maintain good sleep hygiene (regular exercise, healthy diet, managed substance use).

2. Maintaining Healthy Sleep Thoughts:

Continue practicing the cognitive skills you developed.

- **Monitor your thoughts:** Stay aware of your thoughts and beliefs about sleep.

- **Challenge unhelpful thoughts:** If you notice negative thoughts creeping back in, use cognitive restructuring to challenge them.

- **Practice acceptance:** Accept that sleep is variable and that occasional bad nights are normal.

3. Managing Stress and Arousal:

Since stress is a major trigger for insomnia, effective stress management is crucial for long-term sleep health.

- **Regular Relaxation Practice:** Continue practicing relaxation and mindfulness techniques regularly (e.g., a few times a week).

- **Constructive Worry:** Use the Constructive Worry technique to manage worry and problem-solving during the day.

- **Healthy Coping Strategies:** Develop healthy ways to cope with stress (e.g., exercise, socializing, hobbies).

4. Planning for High-Risk Situations:

Develop a plan for managing the high-risk situations you identified.

- *Example:* If you know you have a stressful period coming up at work:

  o Prioritize sleep by maintaining your schedule strictly.

  o Increase your relaxation practice.

  o Be prepared to use Stimulus Control if needed.

  o Use cognitive restructuring to manage anxiety.

By having a plan in place, you will feel more confident and prepared to handle challenges.

Strategies for managing the return of insomnia symptoms

If you notice the early warning signs of insomnia returning, it is important to act quickly. The sooner you intervene, the easier it will be to get back on track.

The "CBT-I Fire Drill":

Think of this as a fire drill. You know what to do when the alarm sounds.

Step 1: Identify the Problem and the Cause:

Acknowledge that your sleep is deteriorating. Identify any potential triggers (stress, changes in routine).

Step 2: Re-implement the Core CBT-I Strategies (The Booster Shot):

Immediately return to strict adherence to the CBT-I principles.

- **Tighten your schedule:** Ensure your wake time is consistent. You might need to temporarily restrict your time in bed (Sleep Restriction) to increase sleep drive.

- **Reinforce Stimulus Control:** Be diligent about getting out of bed if you are awake.

- **Address Cognitive Arousal:** Use the Thought Record to identify and challenge unhelpful thoughts.

Step 3: Monitor your Progress (Use the Sleep Diary):

Start tracking your sleep using the Sleep Diary again for a week or two. This will help you monitor your progress and adjust your strategies.

Step 4: Be Patient and Persistent:

It might take a few days or weeks to get your sleep back on track. Be patient and persistent. Trust the skills you have learned.

When to Seek Professional Help:

If you have tried to implement the CBT-I strategies but your sleep does not improve within a few weeks, or if the insomnia is severe and interfering with your functioning, consider seeking professional help.

- **CBT-I Therapist:** A behavioral sleep medicine specialist can provide personalized guidance and support.

- **Healthcare Provider:** Consult with your doctor to rule out any underlying medical conditions.

Seeking help is not a sign of failure. It is a proactive step toward taking care of your health.

Final thoughts on maintaining healthy sleep for life

You have completed a comprehensive journey through the science and practice of Cognitive Behavioral Therapy for Insomnia. You now possess a powerful toolkit of evidence-based strategies to improve your sleep and quality of life.

The journey has likely been challenging. You have faced discomfort and uncertainty. But you have persevered.

As you move forward, remember these key principles:

- **Sleep is a natural process:** You cannot force sleep. Your role is to create the conditions that allow sleep to occur naturally.

- **Consistency is key:** Maintaining healthy sleep requires consistent effort and practice.

- **Be realistic:** Aim for progress, not perfection. Accept that sleep varies.

- **Be compassionate:** Be kind to yourself during difficult times.

- **Trust your skills:** You have the tools to manage your sleep. Trust your ability to use them.

Healthy sleep is a lifelong journey. By prioritizing your sleep and practicing the skills you have learned, you can enjoy the benefits of restorative sleep and improved quality of life for years to come.

Workbook Activity: Personal Relapse Prevention Plan

This activity will help you consolidate your learning and develop a personalized plan for maintaining your long-term sleep health.

(In a physical workbook, this section would include a structured worksheet.)

Part 1: My Progress and Achievements

- My baseline ISI score: _____ My current ISI score: _____

- My baseline Sleep Efficiency: _____ My current Sleep Efficiency: _____

- The most significant changes I have made: (List 3-5 key changes in behaviors and thoughts).
- The benefits I have experienced: (List improvements in daytime functioning, mood, energy).

Part 2: My Long-Term Sleep Plan

- My optimal sleep schedule (Bedtime - Wake Time): _____ to _____.
- My daily routines to support sleep (e.g., exercise, wind-down routine):
- The cognitive strategies I will use to maintain a healthy mindset about sleep:

Part 3: My High-Risk Situations and Triggers

- Situations that might trigger a relapse for me: (List potential triggers).
- Early warning signs of a lapse: (e.g., increased worry about sleep, difficulty falling asleep, slipping back into old habits).

Part 4: My "Fire Drill" (Action Plan for a Lapse)

If I experience a return of insomnia symptoms, I will immediately:

1. **Behavioral Strategies:** (e.g., Maintain wake time, get out of bed if awake, temporarily restrict sleep window).
2. **Cognitive Strategies:** (e.g., Challenge catastrophic thoughts, practice acceptance).
3. **Stress Management Strategies:** (e.g., Constructive Worry, relaxation).

Part 5: My Support System

- People I can talk to for support:
- Professional resources I can use if needed:

Keep this Relapse Prevention Plan handy and review it regularly. You have the plan to succeed.

Long-Term Sleep Health Strategies

- **Review and celebrate progress:** Acknowledge your achievements to reinforce motivation.

- **Identify high-risk situations:** Recognize your personal triggers for insomnia relapse (e.g., stress, illness, travel).

- **Recognize early warning signs:** Identify the early signs of sleep deterioration to intervene quickly.

- **Develop a maintenance plan:** Create a long-term plan for maintaining healthy sleep behaviors, thoughts, and stress management strategies.

- **Plan for high-risk situations:** Develop proactive strategies for managing anticipated challenges.

- **Implement the "CBT-I Fire Drill":** If symptoms return, immediately re-implement the core CBT-I strategies.

- **Seek help if needed:** Do not hesitate to seek professional help if insomnia persists.

Appendix: Glossary of Terms

- **Adenosine:** A neurotransmitter that accumulates during wakefulness and promotes sleepiness.

- **Automatic Negative Thoughts (ANTs):** Reflexive, rapid thoughts that contribute to negative emotions.

- **CBT-I (Cognitive Behavioral Therapy for Insomnia):** A structured program that helps identify and replace thoughts and behaviors that cause or worsen insomnia with habits that promote sound sleep.

- **Circadian Rhythm:** The internal biological clock that regulates the sleep-wake cycle over a roughly 24-hour period.

- **Cognitive Arousal:** Mental alertness, racing thoughts, and worry that interfere with sleep.

- **Cognitive Distortions:** Systematic errors in thinking that lead to inaccurate conclusions and increased distress.

- **Cognitive Restructuring:** The process of identifying, challenging, and changing unhelpful thoughts and beliefs.

- **Conditioned Arousal:** The learned association between the bed and wakefulness, anxiety, or frustration.

- **Constructive Worry (Scheduled Worry Time):** A technique for managing worry by containing it to a specific time during the day.

- **Homeostatic Sleep Drive (Sleep Pressure):** The biological need for sleep that builds up the longer you stay awake.

- **Hyperarousal:** A state of heightened physiological and cognitive activation.

- **Insomnia (Chronic):** Difficulty falling asleep, staying asleep, or waking up too early, occurring at least three nights a week for three months or longer.

- **Melatonin:** A hormone that signals to the body that it's time to sleep.

- **Paradoxical Intention:** A cognitive technique that involves trying to stay awake to reduce sleep performance anxiety.

- **Relaxation Response:** A physiological state of deep rest characterized by activation of the parasympathetic nervous system.

- **Sleep Efficiency (SE):** The percentage of time spent asleep while in bed (Total Sleep Time / Time In Bed).

- **Sleep Hygiene:** Practices related to the environment and lifestyle that support healthy sleep.

- **Sleep Restriction Therapy (SRT):** A behavioral technique that involves matching the time spent in bed with the actual time spent sleeping to increase sleep drive and consolidate sleep.

- **Stimulus Control Therapy (SCT):** A behavioral technique that aims to strengthen the association between the bed and sleep by limiting activities in bed.

- **Total Sleep Time (TST):** The total amount of time actually spent sleeping.

References

- American Psychiatric Association. (2013). *Diagnostic and statistical manual of mental disorders* (5th ed.). **American Psychiatric Publishing**.

- Baglioni, C., Battagliese, G., Feige, B., Spinali, D., Hertenstein, E., Nissen, C., Voderholzer, U., & Riemann, D. (2011). Insomnia as a predictor of depression: A meta-analytic evaluation of longitudinal epidemiological studies. *Journal of Affective Disorders, 135*(1–3), 10–19.

- Bastien, C. H., Vallières, A., & Morin, C. M. (2001). Validation of the Insomnia Severity Index as an outcome measure for insomnia research. *Sleep Medicine, 2*(4), 297–307.

- Beck, A. T. (1976). *Cognitive therapy and the emotional disorders.* International Universities Press.

- Benson, H., Beary, J. F., & Carol, M. P. (1974). The relaxation response. *Psychiatry, 37*(1), 37–46.

- Black, D. S., O'Reilly, G. A., Olmstead, R., Breen, E. C., & Irwin, M. R. (2015). Mindfulness meditation and improvement in sleep quality and daytime impairment among older adults with sleep disturbances: A randomized clinical trial. *JAMA Internal Medicine, 175*(4), 494–501.

- Bootzin, R. R. (1972). Stimulus control treatment for insomnia. *Proceedings of the 80th Annual Convention of the American Psychological Association, 7*(Pt. 1), 395–396*.

- Borkovec, T. D., Wilkinson, L., Folensbee, R., & Lerman, C. (1983). Stimulus control applications to the treatment of worry. *Behaviour Research and Therapy, 21*(3), 247–251.

- Chang, A. M., Aeschbach, D., Duffy, J. F., & Czeisler, C. A. (2015). Evening use of light-emitting eReaders negatively affects sleep, circadian timing, and next-morning alertness. *Proceedings of the National Academy of Sciences of the USA, 112*(4), 1232–1237*.

- Cohen, S., Doyle, W. J., Alper, C. M., Janicki-Deverts, D., & Turner, R. B. (2009). Sleep habits and susceptibility to the common cold. *Archives of Internal Medicine, 169*(1), 62–67.

- Drake, C., Roehrs, T., Shambroom, J., & Roth, T. (2013). Caffeine effects on sleep taken 0, 3, or 6 hours before going to bed. *Journal of Clinical Sleep Medicine, 9*(11), 1195–1200.

- Espie, C. A. (2006). *Overcoming insomnia and sleep problems: A self-help guide using cognitive behavioral techniques.* Robinson.

- Finan, P. H., Goodin, B. R., & Smith, M. T. (2013). The association of sleep and pain: An update and a path forward. *The Journal of Pain, 14*(12), 1539–1552.

- Gerritsen, R. J., & Band, G. P. (2018). Breath of life: The respiratory vagal stimulation model of contemplative activity. *Frontiers in Human Neuroscience, 12*, 397.

- Haghayegh, S., Khoshnevis, S., Smolensky, M. H., Diller, K. R., & Castriotta, R. J. (2019). Before-bedtime passive body heating by warm shower or bath to improve sleep: A systematic review and meta-analysis. *Sleep Medicine Reviews, 46*, 124–135.

- Hirshkowitz, M., Whiton, K., Albert, S. M., Alessi, C., Bruni, O., DonCarlos, L., … & Adams Hillard, P. J. (2015). National Sleep Foundation's sleep time duration recommendations: Methodology and results summary. *Sleep Health, 1*(1), 40–43.

- Institute of Medicine (US) Committee on Sleep Medicine and Research. (2006). *Sleep Disorders and Sleep Deprivation: An Unmet Public Health Problem.* National Academies Press.

- Kredlow, M. A., Capozzoli, M. C., Hearon, B. A., Calkins, A. W., & Otto, M. W. (2015). The effects of physical activity on sleep: A meta-analytic review. *Journal of Behavioral Medicine, 38*(3), 427–449.

- Manber, R., Edinger, J. D., Gress, J. L., San Pedro-Salcedo, M. G., Kuo, T. F., & Kalista, T. (2008). Cognitive behavioral therapy for insomnia enhances depression outcome in patients with comorbid major depressive disorder and insomnia. *Sleep, 31*(4), 489–495.

- Mitchell, M. D., Gehrman, P., Perlis, M., & Umscheid, C. A. (2012). Comparative effectiveness of cognitive behavioral therapy for insomnia: A systematic review. *BMC Family Practice, 13*, 40.

- Morin, C. M. (1993). *Insomnia: Psychological assessment and management.* Guilford Press.

- Morin, C. M., & Espie, C. A. (2012). *Insomnia: A clinical guide to assessment and treatment.* Springer.

- Morin, C. M., Hauri, P. J., Espie, C. A., Spielman, A. J., Buysse, D. J., & Bootzin, R. R. (1999). Nonpharmacologic treatment of chronic insomnia: An American Academy of Sleep Medicine review. *Sleep, 22*(8), 1134–1156.

- **Morin, C. M., Vallières, A., & Ivers, H. (2007).**
  Dysfunctional beliefs and attitudes about sleep (DBAS):
  Validation of a brief version (DBAS-16). *Sleep, 30*(11),
  1547–1554. *(Replaces the incorrect 1993 DBAS entry.)*

- Perlis, M. L., Jungquist, C., Smith, M. T., & Posner, D.
  (2019). *Cognitive Behavioral Treatment of Insomnia: A
  Session-by-Session Guide* (2nd ed.). Springer.

- Qaseem, A., Kansagara, D., Forciea, M. A., Cooke, M., &
  Denberg, T. D. (2016). Management of chronic insomnia
  disorder in adults: A clinical practice guideline from the
  American College of Physicians. *Annals of Internal
  Medicine, 165*(2), 125–133.

- Rasch, B., & Born, J. (2013). About sleep's role in memory.
  Physiological Reviews, 93(2), 681–766.

- Riemann, D., Spiegelhalder, K., Feige, B., Voderholzer, U.,
  Berger, M., Perlis, M., & Nissen, C. (2010). The
  hyperarousal model of insomnia: A review of the concept
  and its evidence. *Sleep Medicine Reviews, 14*(1), 19–31.

- Spielman, A. J., Caruso, L. S., & Glovinsky, P. B. (1987). A
  behavioral perspective on insomnia treatment. *Psychiatric
  Clinics of North America, 10*(4), 541–553.

- Spielman, A. J., Saskin, P., & Thorpy, M. J. (1987).
  Treatment of chronic insomnia by restriction of time in bed.
  Sleep, 10(1), 45–56.

- Stepanski, E. J., & Wyatt, J. K. (2003). Use of sleep hygiene
  in the treatment of insomnia. *Sleep Medicine Reviews, 7*(3),
  215–225.

- Stutz, J., Eiholzer, R., & Spengler, C. M. (2019). The effects
  of evening exercise on sleep in healthy participants: A

systematic review and meta-analysis. *Sports Medicine, 49*(2), 269–287.

- Xie, L., Kang, H., Xu, Q., Chen, M. J., Liao, Y., Thiyagarajan, M., O'Donnell, J., Christensen, D. J., Nicholson, C., Iliff, J. J., Takano, T., Deane, R., & Nedergaard, M. (2013). Sleep drives metabolite clearance from the adult brain. *Science, 342*(6156), 373–377.